CONTENTS

INTRODUCTION **6**

BREAKFAST SLOW COOK RECIPES **10**

9PS Tasty Breakfast burritos.. 10

7PS Slow cooker Italian baked eggs 10

7PS Tasteful Eggs benedict.. 11

7PS Apple oatmeal muffins 11

6PS Fresh Broccoli quiche 12

3PS Crestless spinach and mushroom quiche................................... 12

6PS Nice Peach scones 13

5PS Applesauce cranberry oatmeal... 13

3PS Crestless spinach and cheese tarts... 14

7PS Slow cooker breakfast casserole 14

6PS Slow cooker casserole 15

6PS apple pie bread pudding.. 15

7PS Apple Cinnamon Oatmeal: 16

3PS Fresh Breakfast Omelets 17

6PS Slow Cook Red Potato Frittata 17

3PS Tomato and Spinach Quiche 18

5PS Ham and Mushroom Crêpes 19

7PS Granola Fruits and Nuts... 20

3PS Slow Cook French Toast 21

3PS Piña Colada Smoothie 21

3PS Mango-Soy Smoothie 22

3PS Slow Cook Savory Mexican Oats: 22

10PS Maple Hazelnut Oatmeal: 23

7PS Crock Pot Apple Granola Crumble: 24

6PS Slow Cook Apple Pie Oatmeal: 24

10PS Bacon, Egg & Hash Brown Casserole: 25

6PS Hot Chocolate Steel-cut Oatmeal: 26

6PS Pumpkin Pie Steel-cut Oats: 27

5PS Sausage and Sweet Pepper Hash: 27

10PS Banana Pecan French toast: 28

10PS Crock Pot Almond Rice Pudding: 29

11PS Blueberry Nutty Banana Oatmeal:... 30

6PS Delicious Potato Oatmeal: 31

LUNCH SLOW COOKER RECIPES.. **32**

Chicken noodle soup 32

Delicious Slow Cook Beef Stew:... 32

Amazing Thai Chicken Soup: 33

Slow Cook Bourbon Chicken: 34

Protein Chicken Tacos:... 35

Chicken with Lemon and Garlic.. 36

Chicken and Rice Casserole: 36

Honey Mustard Chicken: 37

Slow Cook Chicken Cheese Steak... 38

Taco Bowl with Slow Cooker Chicken and Salsa.. 39
Sweet and Sour Chicken 39
Slow Cook Balsamic Chicken 40
Bean and Potato Soup: 41
White Bean and Chicken Chili: 41
Slow Cook Chicken Teriyaki 42
One Pot Chicken Curry 43
Yummy Chicken Italiano 44
Delicious Sweet Potato Chili: 45
Slow Cook Pumpkin Chili: 45
Apple Butter Pulled Pork: 46
Loaded Creamy Corn Chowder: 47
Chunky Squash and Chicken Stew: 48
Slow Cook Tasty Beef: 49
Cauliflower Fried Rice: 49
Fiesta chicken soup 50
Crockpot Italian chicken 51
Superfood Lunch Soup 51
Brown rice and chicken 52
Slow cooker Zuppa Toscana 53
pulled pork chicken sandwiches with goat cheese 53
Lemon garlic slow cooker chicken 54
Amazing Dijon chicken 54
Arizona chuck wagon beans 55
Crock pot split pea soup 55

DINERS SLOW COOKER RECIPES **57**
Slow cooker Spinach Enchiladas 57
Buffalo Turkey Meatballs: 57
Slow Cooker Beef and Barbeque 58
Delicious Slow Cooker Stew 59
White Cheddar Broccoli Mac & Cheese: 60
Slow Cooker Tacos 61
Mushrooms Beef Tips Over Noodles 62
One Pot Beef Ragu 63
Slow Cook Beef Lasagna 63
Delicious Mexican Meatloaf: 64
Asian Taste Chicken Curry: 65
Slow Cook Beef Chili 66
Chicken with Mushroom Gravy: 67
Italian Chicken and Sweet Potatoes: 68
Delicious Tamari Glazed Chicken: 69
Brown Rice and Chicken: 69
Turkey Lasagna Soup: 70
Beef Bourguignon Stew: 71
Slow Cook Fiesta Chili Supper: 72
Vegetarian Enchiladas: 73
Jambalaya with Chicken and Shrimp: 74
Slow Cook Lasagna Turkey: 75

Delicious Hoisin Chicken...76
Crock pot chicken Chili...76
Greatest Buffalo chicken...77
Slow cooker lasagna...77
Slow cooker veggie chili...78
Cheeseburger soup...79
Italian Pasta Faggioli..79
Slow cooker sweet and sour Chicken..80
Sugary Pork Tenderloin..80
Chicken pot roast...81
Slow cooker tomato soup..81
Adobo Pork carnitas...82
Healthy Black Bean Gumbo..82
Slow cooker sloppy joes with lentils...83
Cheesy spaghetti with turkey sausage..83
Balsamic Glazed Pork...84
Slow cooker Porto Beef...85
Slow cooker Barbacoa..85
Slow cooker beef and cauliflower mash..86
Slow cooker Asian chicken noodles with broccoli...87
Chicken cordon bleu...87
Bacon with Ranch Dressing Chicken...88
Vegetarian lasagna...88
Crock pot cheesy chicken and potatoes..89
Sweet tea glazed pork loin...90
Chicken slow cooker tacos..90
Slow cooker chicken stew recipe...91
Slow cooker cheesy risotto..92
Slow cooker pot roast...93
Slow cooker Asian spiced beans..93
Slow cooker rosemary chicken..94
SOUPS, STEW SLOW COOKING..95
Slow Cooker Taco Soup...95
Slow Cooker Meatball Chili...95
Herbal Turkey and Vegetable Soup...96
Vegetable Chicken Stew..97
Delicious Beef Stew..98
Creamy Chicken Soup...99
Creole Chicken Stew...99
Slow Cooker Lentil Soup...100
Tortilla Chicken Stew..101
Root Vegetable and Lentil Soup..101
One Pot Pea Carrot Soup..102
Lentil & Pumpkin Stew...102
One Pot Vegetable Soup..103
Slow Cook Potato Chowder...104
Delicious Minestrone Soup..104
Slow Cook French Onion Soup..105

Sweet Potato One Pot Soup 106

SLOW COOK SNACKS RECIPES **107**

Delicious Plum Pudding with Fruits 107

Nice Hot Cider Cranberries 108

Healthy Cocktail Sausages 108

Refreshing Herbal Composite 108

Slow Cook Chocolate Pudding 109

Gratifying Strawberry Pudding 110

Sweet Macaroni and Cheese 111

Slow Cook Brown Bread with Raisins 111

Tasty Almond Bread 112

Delicious Cinnamon Flavored Oats 112

VEGETABLES AND SIDES **114**

Vegetable Enchilada Casserole 114

Pasta Free Vegetarian Lasagna 115

Brilliant Raspberry Beets 116

Chestnut Brussels Sprouts 116

Easy Maple Mustard Carrots 117

Savory Cherry Cornbread Casserole 117

Mushroom Pecan Wild Rice 118

Lemon Sesame Kale 119

VEGETARIAN RECIPES **120**

Black Bean Enchiladas with Spinach 120

Squash Soup 120

Pea Soup 121

Mustard Casserole 122

Lentil and Pumpkin Stew 122

Slow Cooker Risotto 123

Sweet Potato Soup 124

Potato Chowder 125

Minestrone Soup 125

French Onion Soup 126

SLOW COOKER COOKING TIPS **127**

INSTANT POT BEEF RECIPES **128**

6PTS Instant pot Mexican beef 128

7PTS Maple Smoked Brisket 128

5PTS Freestyle Spicy Braised Beef 129

8PTS Tender Beef Bourguignon 130

6PTS Freestyle Fast Beef Meatballs 130

7PTS Vegetable Stuffed Peppers with Beef 131

7PTS Pressure Cooker Pot Roast 132

8PTS Grain Free Meatballs and Sauce 133

6PTS Pressure Cooker Texas Red Chili 133

INTRODUCTION

Hello and thank you for taking the time to check out this book!

For many of us, Weight Watchers is the ideal way to help us shed those pounds, and to really get the flab off our bodies. Any time that you go on a new diet plan, one that is healthy and is going to help you to lose weight, you are going to see quite a few health benefits. Gaining weight and following a diet and lifestyle plan that is not all that healthy is going to start wearing you down and can make you feel low on energy, have heart and blood pressure trouble, and can even add to your issues with diabetes and more. A healthy diet like what you will find with being on Weight Watchers is going to help to fix a lot of these problems and can get you in better health than ever before. Some of the health benefits that you are going to see when you choose to get on Weight Watchers includes:

Losing weight

One of the main reasons that people decide to go on the Weight Watchers plan is because they want to lose weight. They may have tried to lose weight in the past or they just started to notice that their weight and their health issues have gotten out of hand. Either way, the Weight Watchers plan is a great method to losing weight in a healthy way. While Weight Watchers is more about changing your lifestyle to be healthier, the weight loss is one of the side effects of their healthier lifestyle. You are adding more activity into your day, you are limiting the unhealthy foods, and you are making changes so that the foods you pick are healthy and wholesome. When all of this comes together, you are going to lose some weight on the plan. Simply by losing some weight, you are going to be able to lose a lot of the health issues that you have been dealing with. You are going to gain more confidence, feel better, and look better in your clothes when you are able to follow this program properly rather than sticking with some of the bad eating and lifestyle choices that you have been enjoying.

Fight off diabetes

If you have a history of diabetes in your family or you are worried about being close to diabetic now, you will need to consider getting on a healthier diet. Diabetes is manageable, but it is tough and you could end up with a hose of other medical issues in the process. All the unhealthy foods that you are eating is what is going to make diabetes a reality for you. All the sugars that you take in from cakes, candies, sodas, energy drinks and more are wreaking havoc on the body. In addition, many processed carbs are found in the American diet and these can cause some issues as well since they are converted into sugars within the bloodstream and raise insulin levels. The Weight Watchers plan works to limit some of these bad foods. Of course you can have them on occasion, but they need to become the exception rather than the normal when you are eating. When you have a bit of sugar or some processed carbs in your die ton occasion, and it is coupled with other foods that are really healthy, you are not going to receive quite as many of the bad side effects.

Lower blood pressure

The traditional American diet is full of lots of saturated fats, sodium, and other things that are really bad on your blood pressure. The typical American is going to take in two to three times as much sodium as their body needs each day and this is going to wreak a lot of havoc on their blood pressure.

Over time, the heart is going to have to work harder to get the blood through as the arteries get tighter and close together, leading to a disaster for the heart. Changing up some of the foods that you consume can help to limit the sodium you are consuming and will add in a few good nutrients that can help to reverse the bad effects in your body.

More energy
Keeping up with our fast paced world can seem like an impossible task. You have to keep track of all your work at home, school, work, and all the other obligations and you may fall into bed at the end of the day and wonder how you were able to keep up with it all. Or you may be one of those people who start to droop a bit after lunch time and have to go out for a soda or an energy drink right in the middle of the day. If this sounds like you, it is time to make some changes in your diet. You are eating foods that are high in calories, but are not giving you the right nutrition or the right vitamins to keep the body moving. Instead, you will receive a high of energy for a short while before coming crashing down and needing to either eat more to keep u the energy, or consume some high sugar products. But with a healthy diet like Weight Watchers, you are able to eat foods that fill you up and provide you with energy that is going to last for hours, rather than a few minutes. These foods are lower in calories but really high in healthy nutrients that the body needs to stay healthy and to keep moving properly. Consider swapping out that high carb lunch or the meal at the local restaurant with healthy food options like a lean protein source and fruits and vegetables and see how energized you are by the end of the day.

Get better sleep
Sleep is so important for your whole body. Sometimes when we stress out too much about the things that are going on around us and we will not take care of our bodies in the process. We will eat unhealthy foods avoid exercising, and sleep may be one of the last things that are on our minds. But without sleep, it is hard to lose weight, or even maintain your current weight, manage your stress, and keep your health in good working order. With the help of the healthier lifestyle that you are going to learn how to use with Weight Watchers, you are going to find that it is easier than ever to get some better sleep. You are providing your body with all the good nutrition and exercise that it needs to stay healthy and this makes it so much easier to reduce your stress, and even turn off some of that inner noise that keeps you up, so that you are able to get the sleep that you need.

Lower stress
Who doesn't have a lot of stress going on around them? It seems that everything is so stressful all of the time. You want to be able to enjoy life, but taking care of kids, worrying about family, running to all those activities, and worrying about how work is going and all the bills can add a lot of stress to your daily life. Most people are dealing with an overabundance of stress in their lives and most of them have no idea how to deal with this stress in a healthy way. While stress may seem like something normal and that you won't be able to get to go away, it is going to cause a lot of issues to your body. Stress can cause headaches, weight gain, bad moods, high blood pressure, and a whole host of other issues. When you learn how to deal with your stress and take care of your body, like you will learn to do with Weight Watchers, you will find that a lot of the health issues that you are dealing with. Sometimes, changing the way that you live your life by making it healthier will make a big difference in your stress levels. There are many healthy foods that can help to alleviate your stress levels; eating unhealthy foods can often make your stress levels go through the roof.

Adding in some healthy exercise is going to release some great happy endorphins into the body that will make you feel good and will reduce the stress. This can all help you to get more sleep during the night so that you aren't feeling so stressed out for not getting enough sleep. By the time that you learn how to use the Weight Watchers program, you will find that your stress levels have gone way down. Dealing with your levels of stress is an important part to staying as healthy as possible. Sure there is always going to be some stress that is going on around us in between taking care of kids, work, school, activities, and other obligations. But a healthy diet and some other skills for relaxation can make all the difference in helping you to lose the weight that you want.

Better immunity
Are you tired of feeling sick all of the time? If someone near you gets sick with anything, are you sure to be the next one in line who is feeling down and out? You may need to make some changes to your diet in order to help out with these illnesses and going on a diet like Weight Watchers is sure to help with these. Those who eat a healthy diet that has a lot of healthy vitamins and minerals are less likely to get sick as much as others do. Your immunity is getting the protection that it needs to stay healthy and to fight off all those bacteria and viruses that are trying to attack your body. So if you are tired of spending so much time in the doctors' office and you want to finally feel your best, you need to get on a diet similar to Weight Watchers and see how well all this healthy food can make you feel. There are so many benefits that you are going to be able to get when you start working with Weight Watchers. You will be able to see changes in your whole life, not just in your weight loss the inches that you lose around your waist. It is worth your time to start checking out a healthier diet, like the one that is provided in Weight Watchers, so that you can start feeling better in no time. When it is time to start taking better care of your health and you know that the best way to do this is through the diet that you are enjoying on a daily basis, you will want to give Weight Watchers a try.

This is a simple diet plan that is easy to follow and still gives you freedom, while also giving you some of the extra tools that you need to really see the results that you are looking for. These are just a few of the benefits that you are going to see when you choose to go on the Weight Watchers diet plan. It has all the healthy options that you need, helps you to learn how to pick the right foods for you, and make it easier than ever to see the results that you are looking for! Don't be fooled by some of the other diet plans that are out there. They will promise to help you lose weight or improve your health, but you will find that they ask you to do things that are hard or really bad for your health in order to lose weight. With Weight Watchers, you will get all the nutrients that your body needs so that you can lose weight in the way that is the healthiest for your body and mind. Slow cooker cooking is one of the best things for anyone who wants to lose weight, but doesn't have the time to make said foods. It's really simple, you just have to do some preparation, and then you'll let it simmer. It's a cinch, and when you're using this combined with the weight watcher's point system, you're in for a treat.

Benefits of Slow Cooking
Slow cooking is gaining more and more popularity nowadays, being a technique that many people use to cook slimming meals. The main reason why you should try slow cooking is that it produces meals that are generally low in fat. The steam involved also kills bacteria while keeping most vitamins and minerals intact.

There are many other reasons why you should try slow cooking, such as:
- It saves energy.

A slow cooker uses a lot less electricity than a rotisserie or oven, so it helps you save energy and manage your electric bill.

- It allows you to buy meat cuts that are difficult to chew.

Slow cooking breaks down the meat naturally, meaning you can actually purchase tougher pork or beef cuts.

- It lowers the risk of burning food.

You're less likely to burn food when you're using a slow cooker and it does not heat up your kitchen.

- It is cheap.

Slow cookers are generally cheaper than most cooking devices. It costs around $30 to $100.

- It is easy to use.

The beauty about slow cookers is that you get to cook your meal while doing other household chores. You can read, watch TV, or clean the entire house while you're waiting for your meal to be ready. You do not have to check every now and then. This book will give you just that. You'll learn of some very amazing recipes out there that you can use in your slow cooker that also fit the Weight Watchers point system. Not only that, you'll find out about what the portion size for everything is, along with how many points each serving is, so you can cook it and then divvy it up for the next few meals. It's really that simple, and all you need to do is follow the recipes in order to generate success with your diet. Let this book help you, and by the end of it, you'll know have all the great Weight Watchers recipes that you can use in order to really kick start your program.

BREAKFAST SLOW COOK RECIPES

9PS TASTY BREAKFAST BURRITOS

Prep time: 10 mins
Cook time: 1 hour
Servings: 4
Points: 9

Ingredients:
- 2 t olive oil
- 1 green pepper, chopped up
- 2 cloves of minced garlic
- 4 egg whites
- 2 T chopped cilantro
- ¼ t salt and pepper
- 4 whole-wheat tortillas
- ½ cup sour cream
- 2 chopped scallions
- 1 chopped tomato
- 2 whole eggs
- ½ cup low-fat cheddar cheese, shredded up
- ½ cup salsa

PREPARATION
1. Heat a skillet and then add in the ingredients, sautéing everything until the veggies are tender and the spices are mixed
2. Put the mixture into your slow cooker, and then let cook on high for about ten minutes
3. Season it to taste, being careful with the salt
4. Spoon about ¼ of the mixture into your tortillas and then serve with sour cream and salsa if you so desire.

7PS SLOW COOKER ITALIAN BAKED EGGS

Prep time: 10 minutes
Cook time: 45 minutes
Servings: 4
Points: 7

Ingredients:
- 2 cups of marinara sauce
- 4 large eggs
- ¼ t red pepper flakes, or more or less to taste
- ¼ cup chopped basil
- ½ cup grated parmesan cheese

PREPARATION
1. Turn on slow cooker to heat it up, and then get a baking dish and put the marinara sauce into their along with the basil

2.   Create 4 wells and put an egg in the middle of each hole, and then put some parmesan cheese and red pepper flakes on top
3.   Let it sit in the slow cooker for about 45 minutes, more for desired doneness
4.   Divide the tomato sauce between four different bowls and put an egg within each one of them.

7PS TASTEFUL EGGS BENEDICT

Prep time: 20 mins
Cook time: 1 ¼ hours
Servings: 4
Points: 7

Ingredients:
- 1 T apple cider vinegar
- 4 slices of low-fat bacon
- ¼ cup reduced calorie mayonnaise
- 1 t squeezed lemon juice
- 2 t unsalted butter
- 1 tomato, quartered
- 4 eggs at room temperature
- ¼ cup plain Greek yogurt
- 1 t Dijon mustard
- ½ t lemon zest
- 2 English muffins, toasted

PREPARATION
1.   Fire up a skillet and fill it up with about water halfway and boil. Put in vinegar, break eggs and put it in boiling water. Cook until white set
2.   Sauté the Canadian bacon and cook the bacon for a minute until warmed
3.   Put the eggs, bacon, and the sauce into the slow cooker, letting it cook for about an hour and then from there put it on each of the English muffin halves. You can put more sauce on top in order to top it.

7PS APPLE OATMEAL MUFFINS

Prep time: 10 mins
Cook time: 1 hour
Servings: 12
Points: 7

Ingredients:
- 2 cut apples, shredded
- 1 cup of cooking oats
- 2 t baking powder
- ½ t salt
- ½ cup milk
- 2 cups all-purpose flour
- 1 cup packed brown sugar
- ½ t baking soda

- ½ t ground cinnamon
- 2 T vegetable oil

PREPARATION

1. Spray a muffin pan with cooking spray
2. Mix in all of the ingredients for the muffins together and put them in muffin cups
3. Bake for at least an hour or so, maybe two, until the center of the muffin is clean.

6PS FRESH BROCCOLI QUICHE

Prep time: 10 mins
Cook time: 2 hours
Servings: 6
Points: 6

Ingredients:

- 1 cup egg substitute
- 1 cup baking mix
- ¼ t ground black pepper
- 20 oz., of chopped spinach or broccoli
- 1 chopped red bell pepper
- 2 cups low fat milk
- 1 t salt
- 2 chopped cloves of garlic
- 1 chopped onion
- 4 oz., of mozzarella cheese

PREPARATION

1. Thaw and drain your broccoli
2. Put the broccoli in a glass pan that fits your slow cooker, and then put half of the onions, peppers, and all of the cheese over that.
3. Put rest of the mixture on top of that.
4. Mix the egg mixture, biscuit mix, milk, salt and pepper, and garlic in a blender until it smooths out
5. Put it in the pan and then place it in the slow cooker
6. Bake it on high for about 2 hours or until everything is cooked and browned
7. Cut into six pieces and then serve when it cools.

3PS CRESTLESS SPINACH AND MUSHROOM QUICHE

Prep time: 5 mins
Cook time: 3 hours
Servings: 4
Points: 3

Ingredients:

- 10 oz. of frozen spinach
- 1 cup chopped artichoke hearts
- ½ cup fat-free cottage cheese
- ½ chopped medium onion
- Salt and black pepper for taste

- Cooking spray
- 1 cup sliced mushrooms
- ½ t olive oil
- 2 t minced garlic
- 3 eggs

PREPARATION

1. Prepare slow cooker
2. Sauté the mushrooms and onions with the garlic, putting in the spinach until liquid is lessened
3. Put the rest of the ingredients together, seasoning to taste
4. Cook for about 2-3 hours on low until everything is tender, or about 1-2 hours on high. Season further to taste if needed

6PS NICE PEACH SCONES

Prep time: 15 mins
Cook time: 2 hours
Servings: 4
Points: 6

Ingredients:

- 2/3 of a cup of all-purpose flour
- ½ t baking powder
- A dash of salt
- 1/3 cup low-fat vanilla yogurt
- Cooking spray
- 1 t sugar
- 2 T sugar
- ¼ baking soda
- 1 T chilled butt, cut into pieces
- 2 T chopped dried peach
- ½ t non-fat milk

PREPARATION

1. Put the dry ingredients together into a bowl
2. Cut the butter until it is a coarse meal, putting the yogurt and peaches into the flour mixture, stirring until it is moistened
3. Create a dough and knead a few times. It might be sticky, but that's fine
4. Pat the dough onto a baking sheet, creating some edges
5. Put milk over it and some sugar on top
6. Put these in your slow cooker and cook for the time allotted,
7. At the very end, put them in the oven for about 5 minutes to help raise them.

5PS APPLESAUCE CRANBERRY OATMEAL

Prep time: 2 mins
Cook time: 20 mins
Servings: 1
Points: 5

Ingredients:
- 3 T uncooked oatmeal
- ½ cup applesauce
- 1/8 t ground cinnamon
- 1 T dried cranberries
- ½ cup water

PREPARATION

1. Mix in all of the **ingredients**
2. Pour this into your slow cooker and cook it on high for about 20 minutes, longer if necessary

3PS CRESTLESS SPINACH AND CHEESE TARTS

Prep time: 25 mins
Cook time: 2 hours
Servings: 12
Points: 3 points per tart

Ingredients:
- 1 cup of chopped onion
- 1 cup of roasted red pepper, chopped
- 2 large eggs
- 1 cup reduced fat baking mix
- 2 T chopped basil leaves
- ¼ t black pepper to taste
- 1 t minced garlic
- 5 oz. baby spinach
- 1 cup low-fat milk
- 1 cup shredded mozzarella cheese
- ½ t salt to taste
- ¼ cup grated parmesan cheese

PREPARATION

1. Spray a muffin pan with cooking spray
2. Sauté the veggies until they're well-cooked and the spinach is wilted
3. Whisk the eggs and milk together and then mix in everything else
4. Divide all of these into the muffin cups
5. Bake it for at least an hour or two on high
6. At the last 15 minutes sprinkle a bit of parmesan cheese on top of it and then let it cook for the rest of the time, serving immediately.

7PS SLOW COOKER BREAKFAST CASSEROLE

Prep time: 20 mins
Cook time: 4 hours
Servings: 6
Points: 7

Ingredients:
- 1 pound of frozen hash brown potatoes

- 1 cup shredded low fat cheddar cheese
- 1 cup milk
- ½ t pepper and salt
- ½ pound cooked turkey sausage
- 8 eggs

PREPARATION

1. Brown your sausage and then drain to set aside
2. Grease your slow cooker and then put a third of the potatoes in there, then a third of the sausage, and then the third of the cheese, repeating this for the rest of the layers
3. Beat the rest of the ingredients in a bowl and put it over the ingredients in the slow cooker
4. Cook it on low for at least 4-5 hours or until its set and lightly browned. Cut and then serve.

6PS SLOW COOKER CASSEROLE

Prep time: 20 mins
Cook time: 6 hours
Servings: 6
Points: 6

Ingredients:

- 1 package frozen hash browns
- 1 cup shredded cheese
- 1 package diced mushrooms
- 1 cup milk
- 1 t salt
- ½ t pepper
- ½ t dry mustard
- ½ pound of lean turkey or chicken breakfast sausage
- 1 diced bell pepper
- 14 egg whites
- 6 diced scallions
- `1 t garlic powder
- ½ t paprika

PREPARATION

1. Cover a crock pot with cooking spray, and then proceed to put the bell pepper, onions, mushrooms, and about ½ a cup of the cheese into the crock pot, using about 2-3 layers
2. Put the rest of the shredded cheese on top
3. In a bowl, whisk the eggs with the rest of the spices and put it over the rest of the mixture
4. Cover this up and then cook it for about 6-8 hours or until it's completely cooked through.

6PS APPLE PIE BREAD PUDDING

Prep time: 10 mins
Cook time: 6

Servings: 6

Points: 6

Ingredients:

- 12 slices of low-calorie white bread, torn into small pieces
- 1 cup unsweetened apple juice
- Sugar substitute that equals about ½ cup sugar
- cups of cooking apples, chopped up
- ½ cup diet lemon-lime soda
- 2 t apple pie spice

PREPARATION

1. Cover your slow cooker with cooking spray
2. Put the apples and bread in there
3. In a bowl, mix the rest of the ingredients together until combined
4. Put this over the bread mixture and then mix it to combine
5. Cook it for about 6 hours on low, or until you feel it is done. You can mix it once more before you serve.

7PS APPLE CINNAMON OATMEAL:

Serving Size: 1 cup

Servings per Recipe: 2

Smart Points per Serving: 7

Calories: 205

Cooking Time: 8 Hours

Ingredients:

- A cup outdated oats
- 1/2 teaspoon ground cinnamon
- 1/2 teaspoon vanilla concentrate
- Salt to taste
- 2 cups water to fill Slow Cooker around 1/4 of the way full
- 1/2 little apple, slashed
- Foul sweetener of decision, to taste

Nutrition Information:

Saturated Fat: 0.5 g

Cholesterol: 0 mg

Sodium: 170 mg

Carbohydrates: 27 g

Dietary Fiber: 3 g

Sugars: 12 g

Protein: 3 g

PREPARATION

1. In a small oven-proof bowl, blend together oats, cinnamon, vanilla, and salt.
2. The apples can likewise be included here.
3. Pour two cups water over oats.
4. Fill Slow Cooker around 1/4 to 1/2 of the path full with water (this will rely on upon the span of your Slow Cooker).
5. Include the heatproof bowl with the oat blend to the slow cooker.

6. The bowl with the oats/cinnamon/vanilla has water in it and furthermore sits in the slow cooker encompassed by water.
7. The water level ought to rise practically to the highest point of the bowl.
8. Turn Slow Cooker on low for 7-8 hours overnight. Utilizing a huge spoon, expel bowl from Slow Cooker.
9. Mix in slashed apple and sweetener of choice.

3PS FRESH BREAKFAST OMELETS

Smart Points: 3
Servings: 2
Nutritional Info (per serving):
Calories 110
Sodium 436 mg
Carbohydrates 1 g
Total Fat 6 g
Saturated Fat 2 g
Cholesterol 213 mg
Protein 12 g
Calcium 29 mg
Ingredients:
- 2 eggs, plus 3 egg whites
- 1/2 teaspoon of olive oil
- 1/4 teaspoon each of salt and ground pepper
- 1 tablespoon of water

PREPARATION
1. In a bowl, beat the eggs, egg whites, salt, pepper, and water until frothy.
2. Heat half of the oil in a skillet over medium heat. Pour half of the egg mixture.
3. Cook for a couple of minutes, while lifting the edges using a spatula every once in a while. Fold into a half.
4. Turn the heat to low and continue cooking for a minute.
5. Repeat the process for the rest of the egg mixture.

6PS SLOW COOK RED POTATO FRITTATA

Smart Points: 6
Servings: 4
Nutritional Info (1/4 of the recipe):
Calories 273
Sodium 491 mg
Carbohydrates 30 g
Total Fat 11 g
Saturated Fat 5 g
Cholesterol 203 mg
Protein 16 g
Calcium 172 mg
Ingredients:
- 4 eggs, plus 4 egg whites

- 3 small red potatoes (thinly sliced)
- 4 scallions (thinly sliced)
- 1/2 cup of low-fat (1%) milk
- 1 tablespoon of unsalted butter
- 1/4 teaspoon of ground pepper
- 1/4 cup of shredded fontina cheese
- 1/2 teaspoon of salt
- 2 teaspoons of minced fresh thyme (or 1/2 teaspoon of dried)

PREPARATION

1. Put the milk, eggs, egg whites, cheese, and thyme in a bowl. Mix until well-combined. Set aside.

2. Spray a skillet with a nonstick spray. Set it over medium heat. Put the potatoes, and season with salt and pepper. Cook for 8 minutes while stirring occasionally. Transfer to a plate.

3. Melt the butter in the same skillet over medium-low heat. Cook for 10 minutes or until the bottom is firm.

4. Put the skillet in a preheated broiler and broil it 5 inches from the heat. Do this for 5 minutes or until the center of the frittata is firm. Slice into 4 and serve while hot.

3PS TOMATO AND SPINACH QUICHE

Smart Points: 3
Servings: 6
Nutritional Info (1/6 of the quiche):
- Calories 279
- Sodium 571 mg
- Carbohydrates 38 g
- Total Fat 9 g
- Saturated fat 3 g
- Cholesterol 80 mg
- Protein 14 g
- Calcium 250 mg
- Fiber 3 g

Ingredients:
- 2 eggs, plus 1 egg white (lightly beaten)
- 3 medium onions (chopped)
- 3/4 cup of evaporated fat-free milk
- 1 10-ounce package of refrigerated pizza dough
- 1 10-ounce package of frozen chopped spinach (thawed and squeezed dry)
- 2 teaspoons of extra-virgin olive oil
- 1 teaspoon of sugar
- 1/8 teaspoon each of freshly ground pepper and nutmeg
- 1/2 teaspoon of salt
- 1/2 cup shredded reduced-fat Monterey Jack cheese
- 12 cherry tomatoes (halved)
- 2 garlic cloves (minced)
- 1/4 cup of light sour cream

PREPARATION

1.   Heat oil in a skillet over medium heat. Put the garlic, onions, and sugar. Cook for 10 minutes while stirring occasionally. Put the spinach and cook for a couple of minutes. Remove from the stove. Allow to cool for 10 minutes.

2.   Spread the dough on a floured surface. Shape it into 4-inch round. Loosely cover with plastic and leave for 10 minutes. Roll the dough and fit it into a pie plate. Fold the edges.

3.   In a bowl, whisk the eggs, egg white, milk, salt, pepper, nutmeg, and sour cream.

4.   Sprinkle the cheese all over the crust. Follow it with the spinach mixture and add the egg mixture. Place the tomato halves with the cut part facing side up. Bake in a preheated oven at 350 degrees for 45 minutes.

5.   Allow to cool for 10 minutes before slicing.

5PS HAM AND MUSHROOM CRÊPES

Smart Points: 5
Servings: 6
Nutritional Info (1 crêpe with filling):
- Calories 203
- Sodium 743 mg
- Carbohydrates 19 g
- Total Fat 7 g
- Saturated Fat 3 g
- Cholesterol 87 mg
- Protein 16 g
- Calcium 216 mg
- Fiber 1 g

Ingredients:
- 2 eggs
- 1/2 cup of all-purpose flour
- 3/4 cup of low-fat (1%) milk
- 1/4 teaspoon of salt

For the filling
- 5 tablespoons of dry sherry
- 3/4 cup each of reduced-sodium chicken broth and low-fat (1%) milk
- Freshly ground pepper
- 3 tablespoons of all-purpose flour
- 1/2 cup freshly grated Parmesan cheese
- 2 cups of cremini mushrooms (sliced)
- 3 garlic cloves (minced)
- 2 tablespoons of parsley (chopped)
- 6 slices of deli-sliced cooked lean ham
- 1/4 teaspoon of salt
- 1/8 teaspoon each of cayenne and nutmeg

PREPARATION

1.   Make the crêpes. Combine the salt and flour in a bowl. In another bowl, whisk the eggs and milk. Gradually combine the two mixtures until smooth. Leave for 15 minutes.

2.   Spray a skillet with non-stick cooking spray and put over medium heat. Stir the batter a little. Pour 1/4 of the batter into the skillet. Tilt the skillet to form a thin and even crêpe. Cook for a couple of minutes or until the bottom is golden and the top is set. Flip and cook for 20 seconds. Transfer to a plate.

3.   Repeat the steps with the remaining batter. Loosely cover the cooked crêpes with plastic wrap.

4.   Make the filling. Put the following in a saucepan over medium heat – flour, milk, cayenne, nutmeg, pepper, and 3 tablespoons of sherry. Constantly whisk until thick or around 7 minutes. Remove from the stove. Stir in a tablespoon of parsley and cheese. Loosely cover to keep warm.

5.   Spray a skillet with non-stick cooking spray and put over medium heat. Cook the garlic and mushrooms. Season with salt. Cook for 6 minutes or until the mushrooms are soft. Add 2 tablespoons of sherry. Cook for a couple of minutes. Remove from the stove. Add the remaining parsley and stir.

6.   Put the crêpes side by side on a flat surface. Put a slice of ham in the middle of each piece. Spread a tablespoon of the sauce and 2 tablespoons of the cooked mushrooms. Roll up the crêpes and transfer them to a greased baking dish. Pour the rest of the sauce on top. Bake in a preheated oven at 450 degrees for 15 minutes.

7PS GRANOLA FRUITS AND NUTS

Smart Points: 7
Servings: 12
Nutritional Info (per 1/2 cup serving):
- Calories 296
- Sodium 54 mg
- Carbohydrates 52 g
- Total Fat 8 g
- Saturated Fat 1 g
- Cholesterol 0 mg
- Protein 7 g
- Calcium 48 mg
- Fiber 5 g

Ingredients:
- 1 cup each of dried cranberries and golden raisins
- 6 tablespoons of maple syrup
- 4 cups of old-fashioned rolled oats
- 2 tablespoons each of canola oil and warm water
- 1 teaspoon each of vanilla extract and cinnamon
- 1/4 cup of sesame seeds
- 1/4 teaspoon of salt
- 1/3 cup of honey
- 1/2 cup of slivered almonds
- 1/8 teaspoon of nutmeg

PREPARATION

1.   In a bowl, mix the sesame seeds, nutmeg, almonds, oats, salt, and cinnamon.
2.   In another bowl, mix the oil, water, vanilla, honey, and syrup. Gradually pour the mixture into the oats mixture. Toss to combine. Spread the mixture into a greased jelly-roll pan. Bake in a preheated oven at 300 degrees for 55 minutes. Stir and break the clumps every 10 minutes.
3.   Once you get it from the oven, stir the cranberries and raisins. Allow to cool. This will last for a week when stored in an airtight container and up to a month when stored in the fridge.

3PS SLOW COOK FRENCH TOAST

Smart Points: 3
Servings: 2
Nutritional Info (1 slice):
- Calories 131
- Sodium 244 mg
- Carbohydrates 15 g
- Total Fat 4 g
- Saturated Fat 1 g
- Cholesterol 107 mg
- Protein 10 g
- Calcium 55 mg
- Fiber 2 g

Ingredients:
- 1 egg, plus 2 egg whites
- 2 slices of firm whole wheat bread
- A pinch of cinnamon
- 2 tablespoons of fat-free milk
- 1/4 teaspoon of vanilla extract

PREPARATION
1.   In a shallow dish, beat the milk, cinnamon, vanilla, egg, and egg whites. Soak each slice of bread into the mixture.
2.   Grease a skillet with a butter-flavored non-stick spray over medium heat. Once hot, cook the bread slices until both sides are golden brown. Cook each side for about 3 minutes.
1.   Add 1 Smart Point when you serve each slice with 1 ounce of Canadian bacon or top the slices with fresh strawberries and drizzle with a tablespoon of maple syrup.

3PS PIÑA COLADA SMOOTHIE

Smart Points: 3
Servings: 4
Nutritional Info (per 1 cup serving):
- Calories 115
- Sodium 93 mg
- Carbohydrates 24 g
- Total Fat 2 g
- Saturated Fat 1 g
- Cholesterol 2 mg

- Protein 3 g
- Calcium 90 mg
- Fiber 1 g

Ingredients:
- 1 cup coconut water
- 1 cup of low-fat vanilla yogurt (frozen)
- 1 cup of ice cubes
- 1 cup of crushed pineapple in juice (drained)
- 1/2 cup of pineapple juice

PREPARATION
1. Chill the pineapple for at least 3 hours. Thaw at a room temperature for 10 minutes.
2. Put in a blender, along with the ice cubes, coconut water, frozen yogurt, and pineapple juice.
3. Process until smooth. Serve and enjoy.

3PS MANGO-SOY SMOOTHIE

Smart Points: 3
Servings: 4
Nutritional Info (per 1 cup serving):
- Calories 101
- Sodium 8 mg
- Carbohydrates 25 g
- Total Fat 0 g
- Saturated Fat 0 g
- Cholesterol 0 mg
- Protein 2 g
- Calcium 110 mg
- Fiber 2 g

Ingredients:
- 1 cup of cubed mango
- 1 cup of ice cubes
- 1 tablespoon of sugar
- 1 cup of vanilla-flavored soy drink (chilled)
- 1 tablespoon of sweetened lime juice
- 3/4 cup of mango nectar

PREPARATION
1. Put the ice cubes in a blender. Process until crushed.
2. Add the rest of the ingredients. Blend until smooth.

3PS SLOW COOK SAVORY MEXICAN OATS:

Serving Size: 1/2 cup
Servings per Recipe: 4
Smart Points per Serving: 3
Calories: 86
Cooking Time: 4 Hours

Ingredients:

- 1 cup steel cut oats
- 1 cup salsa
- 2 tablespoons new cilantro, cleaved
- 2-1/2 cups low sodium chicken soup, no sugar included
- 1 cup solidified corn, defrosted
- 1 cup red pepper, finely chopped

Nutrition Information:

Saturated Fat: 0 g
Cholesterol: 2 mg
Sodium: 0 mg
Carbohydrates: 16 g
Fiber: 2 g
Sugars: 2 g
Protein: 3 g

PREPARATION

Mix everything together and let it cook for 3 to 4 hours at low temperature.

10PS MAPLE HAZELNUT OATMEAL:

Serving Size: 1-1/2 cup
Servings per Recipe: 4
Smart Points per Serving: 10
Calories: 358
Cooking Time: Approx. 7 Hours

Ingredients:

- 1/2 cups low-fat milk
- ½ cups water
- Cooking shower /spray
- 2 Gala apples, peeled and cut into 1/2-inch solid shapes (around 3 cups)
- 1 glass uncooked steel-cut oats
- 2 tablespoons cocoa sugar
- 1/2 tablespoons margarine, mellowed
- 1/4 teaspoon ground cinnamon
- 1/4 teaspoon salt
- 1/4 glass maple syrup
- 2 tablespoons hazelnuts, chopped

Nutrition Information:

Saturated Fat: 4g
Total Carbohydrate: 62g
Dietary Fiber: 5g
Protein: 9g

PREPARATION

1. Bring milk and 1/2 mugs water to the point of boiling in a pot over medium-high warmth, blending oftentimes.
2. Coat a 3 1/2-quart electric moderate cooker with a cooking splash.

3.   Put hot milk batter, apple, and next 5 fixings in moderate cooker; mix well.
4.   Cover and cook on low for 7 hours or until oats are delicate.
5.   Spoon cereal into dishes; beat with maple syrup and hazelnuts.

7PS CROCK POT APPLE GRANOLA CRUMBLE:

Serving Size: 1-1/2 cup
Servings per Recipe: 4
Smart Points per Serving: 7
Calories: 180
Cooking Time: 4 Hours and 15 minutes

Ingredients:

- 2 green apples
- 1 measure of your most loved granola grain (you can blend two or types of granola if you wish to)
- 1/8 cup maple syrup
- 1/4 cup squeezed apple
- 2 tablespoons dairy free spread
- 1 teaspoon ground cinnamon
- 1/2 teaspoon ground nutmeg

Nutrition Information:

Total Fat: 5g
Cholesterol: 0mg
Sodium: 135mg
Carbohydrate: 31g
Dietary Fiber: 5g
Sugar: 11g
Protein: 5g

PREPARATION

1.   Peel, center and cut the apples into thick cuts and afterward lumps.
2.   Slice the apple down the middle - then half again and after that those parts in halves as well.
3.   This gives you 8 thick cuts. Cut those thick cuts in lumps around 3 for every cut.
4.   Add everything to the slow cooker and blend well.
5.   Cover and cook on low 4 hours.

6PS SLOW COOK APPLE PIE OATMEAL:

Serving Size: 1
Servings per Recipe: 5
Smart Points per Serving: 6
Calories: 180
Cooking Time: Approx. 8 Hours

Ingredients:

- 1 cup of Steel-Cut Oats (ensured without gluten if vital)
- 4 cups of unsweetened Almond Milk (ensured without gluten if vital)
- 2 medium Apples, slashed

- 1 teaspoon Coconut Oil
- 1 teaspoon Cinnamon
- 1/4 teaspoon Nutmeg
- 2 tablespoon Maple Syrup
- Sprinkle of Lemon Juice

Nutrition Information:

Total Fat: 5g

Cholesterol: 0mg

Sodium: 135mg

Carbohydrate: 31g

Dietary Fiber: 5g

Sugar: 11g

Protein: 5g

PREPARATION

1. Add all the ingredients to your cooking pan. Mix them well by stirring.
2. Cook on low flame for 8 hours or on high flame for 4 hours.
3. Give it a decent stir. Add toppings of your most loved garnishes. Such as peanut butter or crunched up apples.
4. Stash leftovers in the freezer for up to a week.
5. To warm the food, include a sprinkle of almond milk and reheat in the microwave or stove.

10PS BACON, EGG & HASH BROWN CASSEROLE:

Serving Size: 1 cup

Servings per Recipe: 8

Smart Points per Serving: 10

Calories: 342

Cooking Time: Approx. 4 to 8 Hours

Ingredients:

- 20-ounce pack solidified hash
- 8 cuts thick-cut bacon, cooked and coarsely slashed
- 8 ounces destroyed cheddar
- 6 green onions, cut thin
- 12 eggs
- 1/2 glass drain
- 1/2 teaspoon salt
- 1/4 teaspoon pepper
- Cooking oil

Nutrition Information:

Total Fat: 22g

Sodium: 648mg

Carbohydrate: 14g

Dietary Fiber: 2g

Sugar: 2g

Protein: 21g

PREPARATION

1.   Softly oil your moderate cooker with cooking oil.
2.   Layer half of the hash tans into the base and top with a large portion of the bacon, a large portion of the cheddar, and 33% of the green onions.
3.   Put aside some bacon and green onion for, topping and after that rehash with a moment layer of hash cocoa, bacon, cheddar, and onion.
4.   In a substantial bowl, whisk together eggs, drain, salt, and pepper and gradually pour over top.
5.   Cook until eggs are set, roughly 2-3 hours on high, or 4-5 hours on low.
6.   Sprinkle remaining bacon and onions on top and serve promptly, with or without hot sauce.

6PS HOT CHOCOLATE STEEL-CUT OATMEAL:

Serving Size: 1 cup
Servings per Recipe: 4
Smart Points per Serving: 6
Calories: 126
Cooking Time: Approx. 2 Hours

Ingredients:

- 1 cup steel-cut oats
- 4 cup water
- 1/2 cup coconut milk
- 1 tablespoon cocoa powder
- 1 teaspoon vanilla
- 1/4 teaspoon salt
- 1 tablespoon coconut palm sugar or immaculate maple syrup
- 8 drops fluid stevia

Nutrition Information:

Saturated Fat: 6.4 g
Cholesterol: 0 mg
Sodium: 160 mg
Carbohydrates: 12.4 g
Dietary Fiber: 2.1 g
Sugars: 4.4 g
Protein: 2.7 g

PREPARATION

1.   In a substantial bowl, consolidate the water, milk, vanilla, and stevia.
2.   Speed in the cocoa, sugar, and salt.
3.   At long last, blend in the oats. Oil within your moderate cooker.
4.   Pour in the above blend.
5.   Set the slow cooker low for 1-2 hours, and swing it to keep warm before resigning to bed.
6.   In the morning, put everything a blend and devour!

7.   Best with some shaved chocolate in case you're feeling truly degenerated!

6PS PUMPKIN PIE STEEL-CUT OATS:

Serving Size: 1 cup
Servings per Recipe: 4
Smart Points per Serving: 6
Calories: 188
Cooking Time: 8 Hours
Ingredients:
- 1 cup steel cut oats
- 3-1/2 cups water (almond or standard drain can be substituted)
- 1 cup canned pumpkin puree
- 1 teaspoon vanilla concentrate
- 1/4 teaspoon salt
- 1 teaspoon pumpkin pie flavor
- 1/2 cup honey or 2 teaspoons vanilla fluid stevia*
- Sweetener can be included amid cooking

Nutrition Information:
Saturated Fat: 0 g
Cholesterol: 0 mg
Sodium: 193 mg
Carbohydrates: 15 g
Dietary Fiber: 2 g
Sugars: 7 g
Protein: 1 g
PREPARATION
1.   Mix all fixings in the slow cooker and cook on low for 8 hours.
2.   Server hot

5PS SAUSAGE AND SWEET PEPPER HASH:

Serving Size: 2-3 cup
Servings per Recipe: 10
Smart Points per Serving: 5
Calories: 131
Cooking Time: Approx. 5 to 6 Hours
Ingredients:
- 12-ounce bundle cooked smoked chicken hot dog with apple, cut into 1/2-inch pieces
- 1 teaspoon olive oil
- 1/2 mugs cut sweet onion
- Nonstick cooking shower
- 1/2 pounds red-cleaned potatoes, cut into 1/2-inch pieces
- 2 teaspoons clipped new thyme or 1/2 teaspoon dried thyme, pounded
- 1/2 teaspoon ground dark pepper
- 1/4 glass lessened sodium chicken soup
- 1/2 glasses slashed green, red, as well as yellow sweet peppers

- 1/2 glass destroyed Swiss cheddar
- 2 teaspoons clipped crisp tarragon or parsley

Nutrition Information:

Fat: 3g

Cholesterol: 24mg

Sodium: 22mg

Carbohydrate: 18g

Fiber: 2g

Sugar: 6g

Protein: 7g

PREPARATION

1. In an expansive nonstick skillet cook wiener over medium warmth around 5 minutes or just until caramelized.
2. Expel from skillet. In a similar skillet warm oil over medium-low warmth.
3. Include onion; cook around 5 minutes or until delicate and simply beginning to cocoa, blending every so often.
4. Coat the base of a 3 1/2-or 4-quart moderate cooker with a cooking shower or line the cooker with a dispensable moderate cooker liner.
5. In the readied cooker consolidate frankfurter, onion, potatoes, thyme, and dark pepper. Pour soup over blend in cooker.
6. Cover and cook on a low warm setting for 5 to 6 hours or on a high warm setting for 2 1/2 to 3 hours.
7. Blend in sweet peppers. In the event that covered, sprinkle with cheddar.
8. In the event that utilizing low warmth setting, swing cooker to high warmth setting.
9. Cover and cook for 15 minutes more. Before serving, sprinkle with tarragon. Utilize an opened spoon for serving.

10PS BANANA PECAN FRENCH TOAST:

Serving Size: 2 slice

Servings per Recipe: 6

Smart Points per Serving: 10

Calories: 273

Cooking Time: Approx. 3 to 5 Hours

Ingredients:

- 12 (1" thick) cuts entire wheat baguette
- 4 eggs
- 3/4 glass almond milk
- 1 tablespoon coconut sugar
- 1 tablespoon vanilla
- 1 teaspoon cinnamon
- 2 tablespoons coconut oil, liquefied
- 2 bananas cut
- 1/2 lemons, crispy crushed
- 1/2 cleaved pecans
- Nonstick cooking shower

- Uncontaminated maple syrup for serving

Nutrient Information:

Saturated Fat: 5 g

Sodium: 173 mg

Cholesterol: 124 mg

Carbohydrates: 42 g

Fiber: 2 g

Sugars: 25 g

Protein: 7 g

PREPARATION

1. Shower a 5-7 quart moderate cooker with a nonstick cooking splash.
2. Organize baguette cuts on the base of the moderate cooker.
3. Whisk together eggs, drain, coconut sugar, vanilla, and cinnamon.
4. Shower over the baguette cuts, making a point to cover each cut totally with the egg blend.
5. In a blending dish, shower banana cuts with new lemon juice, hurling to coat.
6. Put banana cuts on baguettes in the moderate cooker. Shower with softened coconut oil, sprinkle with pecans.
7. Cover and cook on high for 2-3 hours or on low for 4-5 hours, or until cooked through.
8. Cooking times with shift with various cookers so start to check your moderate cooker at the 3-hour stamp and permit to cook just until the bread starts to turn brilliant cocoa around the edges.
9. Shower gently with unadulterated maple syrup to serve.

10PS CROCK POT ALMOND RICE PUDDING:

Serving Size: ¾ cup

Servings per Recipe: 6

Smart Points per Serving: 10

Calories: 366

Cooking Time: Approx. 2 to 4 Hours

Ingredients:

- 2 cups dry long-grain cocoa rice
- 5 cups almond milk
- 1/2 cups raisins
- 3 tablespoons chia seeds, partitioned
- 1 cinnamon stick
- Sweetener if needed

Nutrition Information:

Saturated Fat: 2 g

Cholesterol: 15 mg

Sodium: 51 mg

Carbohydrates: 69 g

Dietary Fiber: 1 g

Sugars: 10 g

Protein: 12 g

PREPARATION

1.   Include the rice, almond milk, raisins, 2 tablespoons of chia seeds and cinnamon stick in the moderate cooker.
2.   Cover and cook on low 3 to 4 hours or high for 1-1/2 to 2 hours, or until rice is delicate.
3.   On the off chance that utilizing unsweetened almond milk, include either 1/2 cups of coconut sugar, maple syrup or honey before expelling from the moderate cooker.
4.   Sprinkle the rest of the chia seeds before serving.

11PS BLUEBERRY NUTTY BANANA OATMEAL:

Serving Size: 1 cup
Servings per Recipe: 6
Smart Points per Serving: 10
Calories: 346
Cooking Time: Approx. 2 to 4 Hours
Ingredients:
- 2 cups of rolled oats
- 1/4 cup of toasted almonds
- 1/4 cup of chopped pecans
- 1/4 cup of chopped walnuts
- 2 cups milk
- 1 egg
- 2 bananas, sliced
- 1 cup fresh blueberries
- 1 teaspoon of ground ginger
- 2 tablespoons of ground flax seed
- 1 teaspoon of cinnamon
- 1/4 teaspoon of salt for taste
- 1/2 tablespoon of baking powder
- 2 tablespoons of coconut sugar
- 1 tablespoon pure maple syrup
- 1 teaspoon pure vanilla extract
- 1 tablespoon butter, melted
- Vanilla yogurt for serving

Nutrition Information:
Saturated Fat: 4 g
Cholesterol: 39 mg
Sodium: 145 mg
Carbohydrates: 45 g
Dietary Fiber: 7 g
Sugars: 17g
Protein: 11 g

PREPARATION
1.   Join the oats, nuts, flax, flavors, heating powder, and coconut sugar in an expansive bowl.
2.   Blend until joined. In a different bowl, beat the milk, egg, maple syrup and vanilla concentrate.

3.   Layer the bananas and blueberries in your moderate cooker pot. Spread equally with the oats.

4.   Pour the milk blend over top and sprinkle with the margarine.

5.   Cook on low warmth for 2-4 hours, until fluid is ingested and the top is gently caramelized.

6.   Serve warm, finished with the yogurt if preferred.

6PS DELICIOUS POTATO OATMEAL:

Serving Size: 1 cup
Servings per Recipe: 6
Smart Points per Serving: 6
Calories: 164
Cooking Time: Approx. 2 Hours

Ingredients:

- 1 cup of steel cut oats
- 2 cups of low-fat drain
- 2 cups of water
- 1 cup ground sweet potato or 1/2 glass cooked and crushed sweet potato
- 2 tablespoons organic sweetener, pretty much to taste
- Honey or 100% unadulterated maple syrup for taste
- Kosher or Sea salt to taste
- 1/2 teaspoon cinnamon
- 1 teaspoon pumpkin pie flavor

Nutrition Information:

Saturated Fats: 1g
Cholesterol: 3 mg
Sodium: 56 mg
Carbohydrates: 45 g
Dietary Fiber: 5 g
Sugars: 14 g
Protein: 8 g

PREPARATION

1.   Combine all ingredients in the cooker, wrap and cook on a low temperature for approximately 2 hours, or until desired uniformity is reached.

2.   Recommend 4-5 quart slow cooker.

3.   If desired, add chopped raisins and nuts.

LUNCH SLOW COOKER RECIPES

CHICKEN NOODLE SOUP

Prep time 10 mins
Cook time: 6-8 hours
Servings: 1 cup
Points: 8

Ingredients:

- 2 pounds of uncooked chicken breasts, cut into small pieces
- 3 t dried thyme
- 1 t salt
- 6 cups low-sodium chicken broth
- ½ t crushed red pepper flakes
- 1 t oregano
- ½ t black pepper
- 1 bay leaf

When finished, add these

- ½ pound whole wheat spaghetti, broken into pieces
- 1 t lemon juice, more to taste
- ½ cup of chopped Italian parsley for serving

PREPARATION

1. Put the veggies and garlic in the bottom, adding the chicken next, and then the spices. Add the stock after that and then the bay leaf
2. Put it in there for 6-8 hours or until everything is tender. You might see some foam, and if desired, scrape it off and get rid of it
3. Cook the pasta separately and then put it into the soup, mixing it before serving. Add more lemon juice if you so desire.

DELICIOUS SLOW COOK BEEF STEW:

Serving Size: 1 cup
Servings per Recipe: 8
Smart Points per Serving: 8
Calories: 274
Cooking Time: 8 Hours

Ingredients:

- 2 tablespoons olive oil
- 1 pound lean hamburger stew meat, cubed in around 1-inch pieces
- 2 tablespoons flour for covering the hamburger
- 1 cup red wine, (discretionary non-alcoholic wine or vegetable juices)
- 5 red potatoes, cubed
- 1 white onion, diced
- 1 cup carrots, sliced/cubed
- 1 cup celery, sliced/cubed
- 1/2 cup mushrooms cut

- 1 cup peas, frozen or fresh
- 4 garlic cloves, minced
- 1/4 cup tomato puree
- 1 tablespoon soy sauce
- 2 tablespoons horseradish
- 2 cups low sodium hamburger juices
- 3 tablespoons balsamic vinegar
- 2 narrows bay leaves
- 2 sprigs fresh thymes
- 1 teaspoon dried parsley
- 1 teaspoon dried oregano
- 1 teaspoon black pepper
- 1/2 teaspoon sea salt

Nutrition Information:
Saturated Fat: 2g
Cholesterol: 37mg
Sodium: 532mg
Carbohydrates: 37g
Fiber: 5g
Sugar: 7g
Protein: 19g

PREPARATION
1. Start by heating oil in a skillet over medium-high temperature.
2. Toss the meat in the flour then add to the cooker.
3. Make them brown on all sides for around two minutes—meat doesn't need to be cooked through, simply get a pleasant covering on it!
4. Add wine and blend it to relax the bits off the base of the dish.
5. Bring down warmth to medium and stew for 5 minutes.
6. Include the meat, container sauce, and all the rest of the ingredients to the slow cooker.
7. Cover and cook on low for 7 to 8 hours, or high for 4 to 5 hours.
8. Expel the inlet leaves and thyme, and serve!

AMAZING THAI CHICKEN SOUP:

Serving Size: 1 cup
Servings per Recipe: 8
Smart Points per Serving: 11
Calories: 269
Cooking Time: 4 to 8 Hours

Ingredients:
- 5 chicken thighs, skinless and boneless
- 6 cups chicken stock, no fat
- 1 (14.5 ounces) can coconut milk (full-fat)
- 1 teaspoon kosher salt
- 1/2 teaspoon black pepper
- 4 teaspoons ground ginger

- 1 teaspoon red curry powder
- 1 (4.5 ounces) can diced jalapeños
- 1 red bell pepper, seeded and diced
- 1 onion, diced
- 3 carrots, sliced
- 1 big potato, cut into little shapes
- Juice of 1 lime
- 1/4 cup crisply chopped cilantro

Nutrition Information:

Saturated Fat: 11g

Cholesterol: 25mg

Sodium: 812mg

Carbohydrates: 24g

Fiber: 4g

Sugar: 6g

Protein: 14g

PREPARATION

1.   Include all ingredients, aside from cilantro, to the slow cooker.

2.   Cover and cook on low 6 to 8 hours or high 3 to 4 hours.

3.   At the point when carrots are delicate and chicken is done, expel chicken and shred with a fork.

4.   Return destroyed chicken and a large portion of the cilantro to the soup.

5.   Mix soup and serve!

SLOW COOK BOURBON CHICKEN:

Serving Size: 1 cup

Servings per Recipe: 5

Smart Points per Serving: 8

Calories: 380

Cooking Time: 4 to 8 Hours

Ingredients:

- 3 tablespoons molasses or nectar
- 1/4 cup ketchup
- 3 tablespoons apple juice vinegar
- 1/4 cup water
- 5 boneless skinless chicken breasts
- 1/2 teaspoon ground ginger
- 4 cloves garlic, minced
- 1/4 teaspoon pounded red stew drops
- 1/4 cup sans sugar squeezed apple
- 1/4 cup (great quality) Bourbon
- 1/4 cup low-sodium soy sauce
- 1 teaspoon Kosher or sea salt
- 1/2 teaspoon black pepper
- 1/4 cup cut green onions, decorate

Nutrition Information:
Saturated Fat: 1g
Cholesterol: 172mg
Sodium: 745mg
Carbohydrates: 17g
Fiber: 0g
Sugar: 14g
Protein: 32g

PREPARATION

1. Put chicken breasts into a moderate cooker.
2. Whisk together all the rest of the ingredients in a bowl then pour over chicken.
3. Cook on low 4-5 hours or high for 2-3 hours.
4. When cooking is finished, evacuate chicken and shred it.
5. Return chicken to moderate cooker and cook on low for an additional 15 minutes.
6. On the off chance that coveted, serve over cocoa rice with green onions on top.

PROTEIN CHICKEN TACOS:

Serving Size: 1
Servings per Recipe: 8
Smart Points per Serving: 11
Calories: 382
Cooking Time: 4 to 8 Hours

Ingredients:

- 1 pound boneless skinless chicken breast
- 3 cups no sugar included salsa
- 1 teaspoon ground cumin
- 2 tablespoons stew powder
- 1/2 cup corn kernels
- 1/2 cup black beans
- 1/2 cup low sodium chicken soup
- 8 entire wheat flour tortillas
- 1 cup destroyed Romaine lettuce
- 1 huge tomato, diced
- 1 cup low-fat grated cheddar
- 1/4 cup diced avocado
- 1/4 cup plain Greek yogurt

Nutrition Information:
Saturated Fat: 4g
Cholesterol: 57mg
Sodium: 1237mg
Carbohydrates: 44g
Fiber: 6g
Sugar: 7g
Protein: 26g

PREPARATION

1. In a slow cooker, include chicken, salsa, cumin, black beans, chili powder, corn, and juices.
2. Cook on low for 8 hours or high for 4 hours.
3. Remove delicate chicken from cooker and shred with a fork.
4. Come back to a moderate cooker and cook for an additional 30 minutes on low or 15 minutes on high.
5. Spoon around 2 tablespoons of destroyed chicken into every tortilla.
6. Beat with lettuce, tomato, cheddar, avocado, and yogurt.
7. Serve and appreciate!

CHICKEN WITH LEMON AND GARLIC

Serving Size: 1
Servings per Recipe: 6
Smart Points per Serving: 3
Calories: 167
Cooking Time: 6 Hours
Ingredients:
- Ground black pepper (to taste)
- Sea salt (to taste)
- Thyme (1 T dried)
- Chicken broth (1 cup)
- Lemons (3 sliced)
- Garlic (10 cloves chopped)
- Chicken breasts (6 fillets, 2 lbs.)

Nutrition Information:
Protein: 30 grams
Carbs: 36 grams
Fats: 2 grams
Saturated Fats: 1.5 grams
Sugar: 0 grams
Fiber 0 grams
Calories: 167

PREPARATION
1. Prepare the slow cooker by spraying the bottom using a cooking spray to ensure nothing sticks. Place 5 cloves of garlic and 1.5 lemons directly on the bottom.
2. Season the chicken as desired before setting it atop the garlic and lemons. Top the chicken with the remaining garlic and lemons before adding in the chicken broth. Cover the slow cooker and let it cook on a low setting for 6 hours.
3. Strain the liquid in the slower cooker and use it to top the chicken prior to serving.

CHICKEN AND RICE CASSEROLE:

Serving Size: 1 cup
Servings per Recipe: 4
Smart Points per Serving: 9
Calories: 327
Cooking Time: 8 Hours

Ingredients:
- 4 (about 1.5 p.) new boneless, skinless chicken thighs or bosoms, cut into pieces of around 1-inch
- 1 tablespoon additional virgin olive oil
- 3 cups chicken stock, no fat
- 2 vast carrots, peeled and cut into 1/2-inch rounds
- 1/2 teaspoon fit or sea salt, pretty much to taste
- 1/4 teaspoon dark pepper
- 2 cups cooked cocoa rice or quinoa
- 1 cup (defrosted) peas
- 1/2 cup ground parmesan cheddar

Nutrition Information:
Saturated Fat: 3 g
Sodium: 833 mg
Cholesterol: 78 mg
Carbohydrates: 36 g
Fiber: 3 g
Sugars: 6 g
Protein: 25 g

PREPARATION
1. In the slow cooker, include the chicken, olive oil, carrots, juices, salt, and pepper.
2. Cover up and cook on low temperature for 6 to 8 hours or on high flame for 3 to 4, or until chicken is done and carrots delicate.
3. Whenever cooked, include pre-cooked rice, peas, and parmesan.
4. Blend to join and keep cooking for 10 minutes.

HONEY MUSTARD CHICKEN:

Serving Size: 1 cup
Servings per Recipe: 4
Smart Points per Serving: 9
Calories: 327
Cooking Time: 8 Hours

Ingredients:
- 4 (1.5 pounds) new boneless, skinless chicken thighs or breasts, cut into chunks of around 1-inch
- 1 tablespoon extra-virgin olive oil
- 3 cups chicken stock, no fat
- 2 substantial carrots, peeled and cut into 1/2-inch rounds
- 1/2 teaspoon genuine or ocean salt, pretty much to taste
- 1/4 teaspoon black pepper
- 2 cups cooked brown rice or quinoa
- 1 cup (defrosted) peas
- 1/2 cup ground parmesan cheddar

Nutrition Information:
Saturated Fat: 2 g

Sodium: 525 mg
Cholesterol: 66 mg
Carbohydrates: 19 g
Fiber: 1 g
Sugars: 17 g
Protein: 14 g

PREPARATION

1.   In the cooker, include the chicken, olive oil, carrots, stock, salt, and pepper.
2.   Cover up and cook on low temperature for 6 to 8 hours or on high flame for 3 to 4, or until chicken is done and carrots delicate.
3.   Whenever cooked, include pre-cooked rice, peas, and parmesan.
4.   Blend to join and keep cooking for 10 minutes.

SLOW COOK CHICKEN CHEESE STEAK

Serving Size: 1
Servings per Recipe: 5
Smart Points per Serving: 7
Calories: 313
Cooking Time: 6 Hours

Ingredients:

- Ground black pepper (to taste)
- Sea salt (to taste)
- Rolls (6)
- Steak seasoning (2 T)
- Garlic cloves (2 chopped)
- Provolone cheese (6 slices)
- Green peppers (2 sliced thin)
- Onion (1 sliced)
- Light butter (2 T)
- Chicken breasts (1 lb.)

Nutrition Information:

Protein: 29 grams
Carbs: 28 grams
Fats: 6.5 grams
Saturated Fats: 1.5 grams
Sugar: 1 grams
Fiber 2.5 grams
Calories: 313

PREPARATION

1.   Thinly slice the chicken into strips before adding it to a bowl and seasoning with steak seasoning, pepper and salt as needed.
2.   Add the butter to the slow cooker before adding in the green peppers as well as the onions and then top it all with the chick.
3.   Cover the slow cooker and let it cook on a low heat for 5 hours.
4.   Divide the results into 6 servings and add the results to each roll before topping with the cheese and toasting for 2 minutes prior to serving.

TACO BOWL WITH SLOW COOKER CHICKEN AND SALSA

Serving Size: 1
Servings per Recipe: 6
Smart Points per Serving: 9
Calories: 391
Cooking Time: 6 Hours

Ingredients:

- Ground black pepper (to taste)
- Sea salt (to taste)
- Lime juice (1 lime)
- Tomatoes (2 diced fine)
- Red onion (1 diced)
- Avocado (1 sliced into 12 pieces)
- Brown rice (1 cup cooked)
- Cilantro (.5 cups chopped)
- Low fat sour cream (.75 cups)
- Shred Mexican cheese blend (6 oz.)
- Black beans (15 oz. rinsed, drained)
- Salsa (16 oz.)
- Chicken breast (1 lb. boneless, skinless)

Nutrition Information:

Protein: 29 grams
Carbs: 40 grams
Fats: 12 grams
Saturated Fats: 3.4 grams
Sugar: 1.2 grams
Fiber 7.5 grams
Calories: 391

PREPARATION

1. Add the chicken as well as the salsa to the slow cooker and let them cook, covered, on a low setting for 6 hours.
2. Combine the pepper, salt, lime juice, onions and tomatoes together in a small bowl.
3. Create each taco as desired before topping with the mixture from the bowl, 2 slices of avocado, cilantro and 2 T sour cream. Serve promptly for best results.

SWEET AND SOUR CHICKEN

Serving Size: 1
Servings per Recipe: 6
Smart Points per Serving: 6
Calories: 241
Cooking Time: 6 Hours

Ingredients:

- Ground black pepper (to taste)
- Sea salt (to taste)
- Corn starch (2 T)

- Garlic (6 cloves minced)
- Soy sauce (.25 cups)
- Lemon lime soda (.25 cups)
- White vinegar (.5 cups)
- Brown sugar (.5 cups)
- Chicken breast (6 fillets, 2 lbs.)

Nutrition Information:

Protein: 21 grams
Carbs: 20 grams
Fats: 2 grams
Saturated Fats: .5 grams
Sugar: 0 grams
Fiber 0 grams
Calories: 241

PREPARATION

1.   Season the chicken as desired before adding it into the slow cooker.
2.   Combine the rest of the ingredients aside from the cornstarch and add it in on top of the chicken.
3.   Cover the slow cooker and let it cook on a low heat for 6 hours.
4.   Take the chicken out of the slow cooker and set it aside before pouring what's left into a sauce pan and then placing it on the stove on top of a burner set to a high heat.
5.   As it is heating, mix the cornstarch together with a small amount of water before adding that to the saucepan. Let the pan simmer and stir thoroughly to ensure it thickens. Do this for three minutes and then let it rest for 1 additional minute.
6.   Top chicken with sauce prior to serving.

SLOW COOK BALSAMIC CHICKEN

Serving Size: 1
Servings per Recipe: 4
Smart Points per Serving: 4
Calories: 191
Cooking Time: 6 Hours

Ingredients:

- Ground black pepper (to taste)
- Sea salt (to taste)
- Balsamic vinegar (.5 cups)
- Portabella mushrooms (10 oz. sliced thick)
- Pears (2 sliced, cored)
- Chicken breast (1 lb.)

Nutrition Information:

Protein: 25 grams
Carbs: 15 grams
Fats: 1.5 grams
Saturated Fats: 2.4 grams
Sugar: 2 grams
Fiber 3 grams

Calories: 191
PREPARATION
1.   Add all of the ingredients to a slow cooker and let them cook, covered, on a low setting for 6 hours.

BEAN AND POTATO SOUP:

Serving Size: 1 1/2 cup
Servings per Recipe: 8 cup
Smart Points per Serving: 8
Calories: 287
Cooking Time: 8 Hours
Ingredients:

- 1 pound Yukon gold potatoes, peeled and slashed (around 3-4 cups crushed)
- 2 jars northern beans, drained and cleansed
- 1/2 cup slashed onions or shallots
- 2 garlic cloves, minced
- 1/2 cup slashed carrots
- 1/2 cup slashed celery
- 2 tablespoons finely slashed new rosemary or 2 teaspoons dried rosemary
- 1/2 tablespoon finely slashed new oregano or 1 teaspoon dried oregano
- 2 tablespoons crisp thyme leaves or 2 teaspoons dried thyme
- 1 teaspoon fit or ocean salt
- 1/4 teaspoon dark pepper
- 1 teaspoon pounded red pepper chips, discretionary, pretty much for heat fancied
- 4 cups low-sodium vegetable or chicken stock
- 1 parmesan skin or 1 (2-inch) piece parmesan, optional*
- 1 tablespoon additional virgin olive oil
- 1 bay leaf

Nutrition Information:
Saturated Fat: 1g
Cholesterol: 2mg
Sodium: 91mg
Carbohydrates: 53g
Fiber: 10g
Sugars: 2g
Protein: 13g
PREPARATION
1.   Add all fixings to the simmering pot and mix.
2.   Allow to cook on low for 6-8 hours or high for 5 hours.
3.   Remove including the parmesan skin or a bit of parmesan includes a considerable measure of appetizing flavor to the soup and serve.

WHITE BEAN AND CHICKEN CHILI:

Serving Size: 1 cup
Servings per Recipe: 12 cup

Smart Points per Serving: 8
Calories: 315
Cooking Time: 8 Hours
Ingredients:
- 2 pounds boneless, skinless chicken breasts, cut into bite on pieces (around 1/2-inch)
- 1 little sweet onion, diced
- 2 cloves garlic, minced
- 2 jalapeño peppers, seeded and diced
- 1 medium Poblano pepper, seeded and diced
- 2 (4 ounces) jars diced green chilies
- 1 teaspoon legitimate or ocean salt, pretty much to taste
- 1 tablespoon stew powder
- 2 teaspoons cumin
- 1/2 teaspoon black pepper
- 1 teaspoon dried oregano
- 1/4 cup newly cleaved cilantro
- 3 (15-ounce) jars cannellini beans
- 4 cups chicken soup, sans fat, low-sodium
- 1/2 cup decreased fat ground cheddar
- 1 cup low-fat sour cream or Greek yogurt

Nutrition Information:
Saturated Fat: 3g
Cholesterol: 69mg
Sodium: 223mg
Carbohydrates: 31g
Fiber: 6g
Sugars: 4g
Protein: 30g

PREPARATION
1. Include all ingredients, with the exception of cheddar and yogurt, to the moderate cooker, mixed well.
2. Wrap and cook on low temperature for 6-8 hours or high temperature for 3-4 hours.
3. The most recent 30 minutes of cooking time, include the harsh cream and cheddar, blend to consolidate.
4. Cover and keep cooking 30 minutes.
5. On the off chance that covered, before serving orderly with sour cream, cheddar, and cilantro.

SLOW COOK CHICKEN TERIYAKI

Serving Size: 1
Servings per Recipe: 4
Smart Points per Serving: 5
Calories: 217
Cooking Time: 6 Hours
Ingredients:

- Ground black pepper (to taste)
- Brown sugar (.25 cups)
- Soy sauce (.5 cups)
- Yellow pepper (.5 sliced thin)
- Red bell pepper (.5 sliced thin)
- Garlic (2 cloves minced)
- Pineapple (16 oz. chopped)
- Chicken breast (1 lb. cubed)

Nutrition Information:
Protein: 27 grams
Carbs: 25 grams
Fats: 2 grams
Saturated Fats: 1 gram
Sugar: 1.7 grams
Fiber 7 grams
Calories: 217

PREPARATION
1.   In a small bowl, combine the brown sugar, black pepper, garlic and soy sauce and mix well.
2.   Add the chicken to the slow cooker before topping with the soy sauce mixture and the pineapple.
3.   Cover the slow cooker and let it cook on a low setting for 6 hours, after 5 hours remove the lid to allow the sauce to thicken.

ONE POT CHICKEN CURRY

Serving Size: 1
Servings per Recipe: 4
Smart Points per Serving: 6
Calories: 272
Cooking Time: 4 Hours

Ingredients:
- Ground black pepper (to taste)
- Sea salt (to taste)
- Cornstarch (1 T)
- Brown sugar (2 T)
- Curry paste (3 T)
- Lime juice (1 lime)
- Garlic cloves (5 minced)
- Coconut milk (15 oz.)
- Stir fry vegetables (16 oz.)
- Yellow onion (1 sliced thin)
- Chicken breast (1 lb. diced)

Nutrition Information:
Protein: 28 grams
Carbs: 17 grams

Fats: 9 grams
Saturated Fats: 2.7 grams
Sugar: 9 grams
Fiber 3 grams
Calories: 272

PREPARATION

1.   Season chicken as desired before adding it to the slow cooker and covering it with the onion.
2.   Combine the curry paste, sugar, garlic, lime juice and coconut milk in a bowl and mix well.
3.   Add the results to the slow cooker and cook, covered, on a low setting for 5 hours.
4.   When there is half an hour of cooking time remaining, mix in the vegetables as well as the cornstarch mixed with 1 T water.

YUMMY CHICKEN ITALIANO

Serving Size: 1
Servings per Recipe: 6
Smart Points per Serving: 5
Calories: 225
Cooking Time: 6 Hours

Ingredients:

- Ground black pepper (to taste)
- Sea salt (to taste)
- Paprika (2 tsp.)
- Chicken broth (1 cup)
- White wine (1 cup)
- Light butter (1 T)
- Cream cheese (8 oz.)
- Italian dressing mix (1 packet)
- Portabella mushrooms (8 oz. sliced)
- Mushrooms (8 oz. sliced)
- Chicken breast (1.5 lbs.)

Nutrition Information:

Protein: 31 grams
Carbs: 9 grams
Fats: 3 grams
Saturated Fats: 5.7 grams
Sugar: 3 grams
Fiber 1 grams
Calories: 225

INGREDIENTS

PREPARATION

1.   Add the butter to a saucepan before placing it on the stove on top of a burner set to a medium heat and mix in the Italian dressing thoroughly.
2.   Add in the chicken broth, wine and cream cheese and keep stirring until the cream cheese has melted.

3.	Add the mushrooms to the slow cooker before seasoning the chicken and adding it in as well.

4.	Add all of the ingredients to a slow cooker and let them cook, covered, on a low setting for 6 hours.

DELICIOUS SWEET POTATO CHILI:

Serving Size: 1 cup
Servings per Recipe: 6 cup
Smart Points per Serving: 8
Calories: 275
Cooking Time: 6 to 8 Hours

Ingredients:

- 1 pound ground turkey
- 1 sweet onion, diced
- 1 jalapeno, seeded and minced
- 3 garlic cloves, minced
- 2 sweet potatoes, cubed
- 1 (14.5 ounces) can dark beans
- 1 (14.5 ounces) fire simmered pulverized tomatoes
- 2 cups low-sodium chicken juices
- 1 teaspoon cinnamon
- 1 tablespoon bean stew powder
- 1 teaspoon cumin
- 1 teaspoon sea salt
- 1/2 teaspoon dark pepper
- 1 tablespoon unsweetened cocoa powder

Nutrition Information:

Saturated Fat: 2g
Cholesterol: 52mg
Sodium: 676mg
Carbohydrates: 33g
Fiber: 9g
Sugar: 8g
Protein: 23g

PREPARATION

1.	Add all ingredients to the slow cooker, separating the ground turkey into bits with a wood spoon.

2.	Blend to consolidate. Boil on low flame for 6 to 8 hours or high flame for 3 to 4 hours.

3.	On the off chance that coveted, present with a dab of sour cream or Greek yogurt and entire grain tortillas disintegrated on top.

SLOW COOK PUMPKIN CHILI:

Serving Size: 1 cup
Servings per Recipe: 6 cup
Smart Points per Serving: 7

Calories: 214
Cooking Time: 6 to 8 Hours
Ingredients:
- 1 onion, diced
- 2 (14 ounce) cans crushed tomatoes
- 2 (14 ounces) cans black beans, a drained
- 1 carrot, shredded
- 1 bell pepper, diced
- 1 jalapeno, veins and seeds removed and minced
- 2 cloves garlic, minced
- 1 1/2 cups pumpkin puree
- 1 cups low sodium vegetable broth
- 2 tablespoons chili powder
- 1 teaspoon pumpkin pie spice
- 1 teaspoon kosher salt
- 1/2 teaspoon black pepper

Nutrition Information:
Saturated Fat: 0g
Cholesterol: 0mg
Sodium: 841mg
Carbohydrates: 43g
Fiber: 16g
Sugar: 11g
Protein: 12g

PREPARATION
1. Add everything to your slow cooker and stir to combine.
2. Cook on low for 5 to 6 hours or high for 2 to 3 hours.
3. Present with a spoonful of Greek yogurt or avocado slices.

APPLE BUTTER PULLED PORK:

Serving Size: 1 cup
Servings per Recipe: 6 cup
Smart Points per Serving: 12
Calories: 352
Cooking Time: 2 Hours
Ingredients:
- 5 apples, peeled, cored and diced
- 2 teaspoons cinnamon
- 1/2 teaspoon nutmeg
- 1/4 teaspoon allspice
- 1/4 teaspoon ground cloves
- 1/4 cup coconut sugar
- 1/4 cup apple cider vinegar
- 3 cloves of garlic, minced
- 1 medium onion, chopped

- 1 tablespoon spicy brown mustard
- 1 teaspoon kosher salt
- 1/2 teaspoon black pepper
- 4 pork loin chops

Nutrition Information:

Saturated Fat: 4g

Cholesterol: 92mg

Sodium: 426mg

Carbohydrates: 33g

Fiber: 5g

Sugar: 23g

Protein: 28g

PREPARATION

1. Place apples, cinnamon, nutmeg, allspice and coconut sugar into slow cooker.
2. Cook on low for four hours, or high for two hours.
3. Add cider vinegar, garlic, onion, mustard, salt, and pepper.
4. Combine the apples, then adjoin pork chops.
5. Wrap the chops with the apple mix. Cook for an additional four hours on low down temperature, or maximum two hours on high flame.
6. Remove pork, shred and return to the slow cooker.
7. Roast on high flame for ten more minutes or so, and then serve!

LOADED CREAMY CORN CHOWDER:

Serving Size: 1 ½ cup

Servings per Recipe: 6

Smart Points per Serving: 9

Calories: 269

Cooking Time: Approx. 4 to 8 Hours

Ingredients:

FOR THE CHOWDER:

- 4 cups vegetable stock
- 2 cups almond milk, unsweetened or 2 cups canned coconut milk (creamier outcomes)
- 2 1/2 tablespoons cornstarch
- 2 tablespoons olive oil
- 1 teaspoon garlic powder
- 1 teaspoon onion powder
- 3/4 teaspoon salt
- 1/2 teaspoon pepper
- 2 cups red potato, diced
- 1 (16-ounce) bundle solidified corn

FOR THE TOPPINGS:

- 1/4 cup diced tomato
- 1/4 cup diced purple onion
- 1/4 cup daintily cut scallions
- 1/4 cup decreased fat cheddar

Nutrition Information:
Saturated Fat: 4 g
Carbohydrates: 34 g
Dietary Fiber: 3 g
Sugars: 8 g
Protein: 10 g

PREPARATION

1.   In a 3-4 quart moderate cooker, whisk together vegetable stock, almond milk, cornstarch, olive oil, garlic powder, onion powder, salt, and pepper.
2.   Mix in potato and corn. Cover up and cook on low temperature for 6 to 7 hours or on high flame for 3 to 4 hours.
3.   Serve finished with your most loved fixings.
4.   For creamier result, expel 2-3 cups of the chowder before serving and add them to a blender.
5.   Puree on high and after that arrival to the soup, blending.
6.   On the other hand, you can embed a hand blender into the soup and puree until covered surface/level of richness is accomplished.

CHUNKY SQUASH AND CHICKEN STEW:

Serving Size: 2 cup
Servings per Recipe: 4
Smart Points per Serving: 8
Calories: 297
Cooking Time: Approx. 4 Hours

Ingredients:

- 15 ounces chicken bosoms, hacked into nibble estimated pieces
- Flour, for covering
- 1/2 teaspoon salt
- 1/8 teaspoon pepper
- 2 tablespoons additional virgin olive oil
- 2 1/2 cups chicken juices
- 1 medium onion, coarsely slashed
- 14 ounces squash, diced
- 1-1/2 cups vegetable juices
- 3 crisp sage leaves, chopped or torn

Nutrition Information:
Saturated Fat: 2 g
Cholesterol: 69 mg
Sodium: 245 mg
Carbohydrates: 21 g
Sugars: 5 g
Protein: 27 g

PREPARATION

1.   Coat the chicken with flour and shake off the abundance.
2.   Over medium warmth, in a pan with additional virgin olive oil, chestnut the chicken then season with salt and pepper.

3.   Try not to stuff. Cook in clusters if necessary. Pour 1 cup chicken soup in the pan and cook until the sauce thickens.

4.   Exchange the substance of the pan to the moderate cooker. Include a smidgen all the more additional virgin olive oil in the pot then sauté the onions over low - medium warmth for around 5 minutes.

5.   Exchange the onions to the moderate cooker. Include the squash, staying chicken stock, and sage in the moderate cooker.

6.   Set on low for 4 hours.

SLOW COOK TASTY BEEF:

Serving Size: 1/10
Servings per Recipe: 10
Smart Points per Serving: 13
Calories: 400
Cooking Time: Approx. 8 Hours

Ingredients:

- 1 (3-pound) meat (round or chuck)
- 1/4 cup additional virgin olive oil
- 1/4 cup crushed garlic
- 1/2 teaspoons ocean salt
- 1 teaspoon pepper
- 1/2 cup veggie or meat soup

Nutrition Information:

Saturated Fat: 11 g
Cholesterol: 124 mg
Sodium: 229 mg
Carbohydrates: 2 g
Sugars: 0 g
Protein: 27 g

PREPARATION

1.   Put meat in a 4-quart cooker. Sprinkle with olive oil, garlic, sea salt, and pepper.

2.   Pour veggie soup around the outside of the meat.

3.   Cover and cook on low for 8-10 hours or on high for 6-8 hours.

4.   At the point when the meat is amazingly delicate, expel it from the slow cooker and shred with a fork.

5.   Serve in tacos, with your most loved sauce and pureed potatoes, mix it into bean stew, cook it into Shepherd's Pie, or top it with teriyaki sauce.

6.   Serve it over cocoa rice.

CAULIFLOWER FRIED RICE:

Serving Size: 2 cups
Servings per Recipe: 4
Smart Points per Serving: 5
Calories: 172
Cooking Time: Approx. 4 to 8 Hours

Ingredients:

- 2 heads cauliflower
- 2 tablespoons ginger-garlic puree (or new garlic and ginger root, peeled and minced)
- 1/2 cup vegetable soup
- 2 eggs
- 1 cup solidified vegetable blend
- 1/2 cup Boars Head turkey ham, diced (discretionary)
- 1/4 cup green onions, diced
- 1/4 cup cilantro (discretionary)
- 2 tablespoons lite (low-sodium) soy sauce or to taste

Nutrition Information:

Saturated Fat: 2 g

Cholesterol: 92 mg

Sodium: 405 mg

Carbohydrates: 22 g

Sugars: 6 g

Protein: 13 g

PREPARATION

1. Cut the florets off each head of cauliflower.
2. Put the florets in an extensive nourishment processor.
3. Beat until finely disintegrated.
4. In an extensive simmering pot, include cauliflower pieces, ginger garlic puree, and vegetable stock.
5. Cover and cook on high for 2 hours or on low for 3-4 hours.
6. 30 minutes prior to plating, beat the eggs together and mix them in a saucepan.
7. Include eggs, solidified veggies, and diced turkey ham (if craved) to the simmering pot.
8. Permit to cook for 30 minutes more, or until the solidified veggies are warm.
9. Mix in green onions and cilantro. Soy sauce to taste.
10. Serve and enjoy!

FIESTA CHICKEN SOUP

Prep time: 5 mins

Cook time: 6-8 hours

Servings: 1 cup

Points: 4

Ingredients:

- ½ cup diced onion
- 1 can black beans and kidney beans, both drained
- 1 can diced green chili peppers
- 3 cups chicken broth, low sodium
- Juice from a lime
- 1 t cumin and chili powder
- ½ t black pepper
- ½ cup chopped cilantro
- 1 clove minced garlic
- 1 can diced tomatoes

- 1 cup corn, frozen or fresh
- 1 T chili powder
- ½ t cayenne pepper
- Salt to taste
- 2 chicken breasts fillets, cut into cubes.

PREPARATION

1. Take all of the ingredients and put them into a slow cooker, cooking this on low for at least 6-8 hours
2. Season to taste and then serve.

CROCKPOT ITALIAN CHICKEN

Prep time: 10 minutes
Cook time: 4-5 hours
Servings: 1 chicken with about a cup of cheese, 6 servings
Points: 8

Ingredients:

- 8 boneless chicken breasts
- 2 cloves mashed garlic
- 1 T Italian seasoning
- 2 cups shredded parmesan cheese
- 2 T olive oil
- 2 cups chicken broth
- Salt and pepper for taste
- 1 carton of drained diced tomatoes

PREPARATION

1. Put the chicken on a cooking rack and put the broth at the bottom of the slow cooker
2. Put the cloves in there, and then put olive oil and the seasonings on top
3. Pour the tomatoes on top of that and then the cheese
4. Cook it for about 4-5 hours on low, serving over zucchini spaghetti if so desired.

SUPERFOOD LUNCH SOUP

Prep time: 5 mins
Cook time: 6-8 hours
Servings: 1 cup, 8
Points: 5

Ingredients:

- 2 cups sliced carrots
- 1 cup frozen green beans
- 1 diced onion
- 2 cans of black beans, drained
- ½ t black pepper
- 1 t cumin
- 2 cups vegetable juice
- 1 sweet potato, cubed
- ½ cup chopped cilantro

- 1 clove of minced garlic
- ½ t red pepper flakes
- 1 t chili powder
- Salt to taste
- 2 cups low-sodium veggie broth

PREPARATION

1. Take all of the ingredients and put them in a slow cooker
2. Cook on low for about 6-8 hours, or until tender
3. If you want, you can add a tablespoon of cheddar cheese on top
4. If you want a less subtle onion taste, sauté the onion in olive oil for about 5 minutes, adding the garlic for another minute and then placing it in the slow cooker with the rest of the ingredients.

BROWN RICE AND CHICKEN

Prep time: 15 mins
Cook time: 3-5 hours
Servings: 1 cup, 8 servings
Points: 7

Ingredients:

For the rice:
- 2 cups brown rice
- 1 can organic diced tomatoes
- ½ large chopped sweet onion
- Organic herb mix without salt, usually about 2 T but more to taste
- ½ t paprika
- 5 cups water
- 4 ribs of diced organic celery
- Sirach hot sauce, whatever to taste
- 1 t cumin

Chicken:
- 4 boneless chicken breasts
- Siracha to put over chicken
- 1 T red chili pepper
- 1 t paprika and cumin
- 2 rosemary sprigs
- ½ cup Yoshida sauce
- Sprinkling of organic herb mix to taste
- ½ t cayenne pepper, more or less to taste

PREPARATION

1. You can do this in separate crock pots if you have them, or you can do it together. If you do it separately, you can help mix it better.
2. If you do it separately, first take the rice and mix it together with the veggies and the spices. You can then put it in the slow cooker and let it cook it for about 3 hours

3.   For the chicken, you can use a large crock pot and let it cook for about 4-5 hours. Cook the chicken by putting everything together and letting it mix. You can open the lid and shred the chicken.

4.   When done, remove the rosemary sprigs.

SLOW COOKER ZUPPA TOSCANA

Prep time: 15 mins
Cook time: 4.5 hours
Servings: 6
Points: 6

Ingredients:
*   1 pound Italian chicken sausage of choice or turkey sausage
*   4 cloves minced garlic
*   3 cups chicken stock
*   2 T whole wheat flour
*   Salt and pepper for taste
*   1 pound Yukon potatoes, diced
*   1 onion, peeled and diced
*   3 cups baby spinach leaves
*   1 cup half and half
*   Red pepper flakes if desired

PREPARATION

1.   Put the sausage, garlic potatoes, and the onions into your slow cooker and put the chicken stock on top of this. Let it cook on low for 4 hours until everything is softened

2.   Whisk the half and half and flour and put it into the slow cooker with the spinach, mixing it. Cook it on high for about 30 minutes or so to help thicken the soup

3.   Season as necessary with the seasonings listed

PULLED PORK CHICKEN SANDWICHES WITH GOAT CHEESE

Prep time: 15 mins
Cook time: 7 hours
Servings: 6
Points: 8

Ingredients:
*   6 sandwich rolls, Panini rolls work best
*   1 jar of roasted red pepper, chopped up
*   6 oz., of goat cheese
*   4 cloves minced garlic
*   Salt and pepper for taste
*   1 pound of boneless, skinless chicken breasts
*   1 package of frozen spinach
*   Cup basil leaves
*   1 package of Italian dressing

PREPARATION

1.   Put the chicken in the slow cooker, and then put in the Italian dressing and the garlic. Put the dressing and garlic well on all sides
2.   Cook it on low for about 5 hours
3.   Shred the chicken and then add in the spinach and red peppers. Cook it again for another two hours, seasoning to taste
4.   Toast the rolls and put the goat cheese on there. Put about ¾ of a cup of chicken and put it onto the buns. Put some basil leaves on top of that, and then the latter half of the bun for best results.

LEMON GARLIC SLOW COOKER CHICKEN

Prep time: 5 mins
Cook time: 6 hours
Servings: 6
Points: 3

Ingredients:
- 2 pounds of boneless, skinless, chicken breasts, cut into fillets
- 3 sliced lemons
- 1 T dried thyme
- ½ t black pepper
- 10 chopped garlic cloves
- 1 cup fat-free chicken broth
- 1 t salt, more for taste

PREPARATION
1.   Coat the bottom of a slow cooker with the cooking spray, putting half of the lemons and the garlic at the bottom of it
2.   Season the chicken breasts with the spices and then put it over the lemon and garlic
3.   Put the rest of the lemon and garlic on top, then the broth over everything
4.   Cook it on low for about 4-6 hours or so, until everything is cooked through. You can strain the liquid and serve it over the chicken if you so desire.

AMAZING DIJON CHICKEN

Prep time: 10 minutes
Cook time: 6 hours
Servings: 4
Points: 7

Ingredients:
- 1 pound of boneless, skinless chicken breasts, ideally 4 small breasts
- 2 pounds of thinly sliced red potatoes
- 3 T Dijon mustard
- 1 T lemon zest
- 1 t salt
- Chopped chives to garnish
- 1 onion, sliced thinly
- 1 cup fat-free chicken broth of choice
- Juice from 2 lemons

- 1 T dried oregano
- ½ t black pepper

PREPARATION

1. Take the chicken breasts and put them in a crock pot and then season with the salt and pepper, along with 1 t of the oregano
2. Put the potatoes and onion on top
3. Whisk the rest of the ingredients together
4. Put it over the chicken, onions, and the potatoes, cooking it on low for about 6-8 hours or high for 4-6 hours
5. Put chives on top of the chicken before you serve it for the best taste.

ARIZONA CHUCK WAGON BEANS

Prep time: 10 minutes
Cook time: 10 hours on low, 6 on high
Servings: 6
Points: 6

Ingredients:

- 1 pound of navy beans, either dried or pinto
- ¼ pound of lean pork loins, diced and boneless
- 1 minced garlic clove
- pounds cubed extra-lean round steak
- ½ t crumbled oregano
- ¼ t ground cumin
- 6 cups water
- 1 chopped onion
- 1 chopped green pepper
- 2 t salt
- ¼ t red pepper
- 8 oz. tomato sauce

PREPARATION

1. Rinse the beans well and then put them in water.
2. Let them boil and cook, and you can then let them stand for a while if desired
3. Brown the pork on each side and then sauté the onion, green pepper, and the garlic in the pan drippings. Put all of this into the slow cooker and then combine the salt, oregano, the red pepper, tomato sauce, and the cumin into there.
4. You can bring more liquid in above the beans if needed
5. Cook it on low for 10 hours or high for 6 hours, until the beans are very tender.

CROCK POT SPLIT PEA SOUP

Prep time: 5 mins
Cook time: 4-8 hours
Servings: 12
Points: 2

Ingredients:

- 1 pound of dried split beans

- 2 ham bones
- 1 T minced garlic
- Light sour cream to garnish
- 8 cups chicken broth
- ½ cup chopped onion
- 1 cup chopped carrot
- More ham bone for serving if desired

PREPARATION

1. Put all of the ingredients into a slow cooker
2. Cook it on high for 4-6 hours, or on low for 8-10
3. Take the ham bone out, and then puree to the right consistency if you want
4. Serve it with some hot sour cream and more ham if you so desire.

DINERS SLOW COOKER RECIPES

SLOW COOKER SPINACH ENCHILADAS

Prep time: 15 mins
Cook time: 3 hours
Servings: 8
Points: 7

Ingredients:

- 1 package of thawed frozen spinach
- 1 cup of corn
- 2 jars salsa Verde
- 2 cups reduced fat sharp cheddar, shredded up
- 1 t ground cumin and coriander
- 1 t chili powder
- 1 can of black beans, drained and rinsed out
- 8 whole wheat tortillas
- ½ cup sour cream
- Juice from a lime

PREPARATION

1. Squeeze water from spinach and then mash the black beans with a fork. Do about half of these, and then add in the rest of the ingredients besides the tortillas and the salsa
2. Put a jar of the salsa into the bottom of your slow cooker and then put the bean and spinach mixture into this, rolling it up and putting it seam-side down. Lay them on a single layer to make it easier with removing
3. Top it with salsa and more shredded cheese
4. Cook it for about 3 hours and top with the sour cream, cilantro, onions, and jalapenos, using other toppings of choice.

BUFFALO TURKEY MEATBALLS:

Serving Size: 3
Servings per Recipe: 18
Smart Points per Serving: 10
Calories: 274
Cooking Time: Approx. 4 Hours

Ingredients:

For Meatballs

- 1/4 cup non-fat milk
- 2 cuts entire wheat sandwich bread
- 14 ounces lean, ground chicken or turkey
- 1 teaspoon salt, partitioned
- 1/4 teaspoon pepper
- 1/4 teaspoon cayenne pepper
- 1/2 cup Parmesan cheddar
- 1 egg

For Sauce
- 2 teaspoons olive oil
- 1 little sweet onions, diced
- 2 cloves garlic, minced
- 1 cup hot sauce
- 1 (4 ounces) can dice green chilies
- 1/2 cup nectar
- 1 teaspoon bean stew powder
- 1 teaspoon paprika
- 1/4 teaspoon cayenne pepper
- 1/2 teaspoon dark pepper
- 1 teaspoon genuine or ocean salt

Nutrition Information:
Saturated Fat: 4g
Cholesterol: 91mg
Sodium: 1630mg
Carbohydrates: 27g
Sugar: 19g
Protein: 18g

PREPARATION
1. Preheat stove to 450 degrees and line a preparing sheet with aluminum thwart.
2. In a little bowl, absorb the bread the milk. In an extensive bowl, blend the chicken or turkey, Parmesan, 1/2 teaspoon salt, pepper, egg, and the bread absorbed milk.
3. Blend well until it gets to be distinctly conservative.
4. Get about a tablespoon of the meat then come in the middle of your palms to make the meatballs—we made them utilizing a 1" scoop.
5. Put them on the heating sheet. Cook for 6 minutes.
6. For the sauce, warm the olive oil on medium-low. Include the onions and garlic and sauté until onions are translucent.
7. Include the onions, garlic, and every one of extra fixings to a bowl and race until smooth.
8. Add enough meatballs to cover the base of the moderate cooker, and then pour half of the sauce.
9. Include the rest of the meatballs and pour whatever remains of the sauce.
10. Cover and cook on low 2-4 hours, or until meatballs are cooked through.

SLOW COOKER BEEF AND BARBEQUE

Serving Size: 2
Servings per Recipe: 8
Smart Points per Serving: 9
Calories: 313
Cooking Time: Approx. 6 Hours

Ingredients:
- Ground black pepper (to taste)
- Sea salt (to taste)
- Cayenne pepper (.25 tsp.)

- Paprika (1 tsp.)
- Garlic powder (1 tsp.)
- Onion powder (1 T)
- Worcestershire sauce (2 tsp.)
- Hot sauce (1 T)
- Brown sugar (.5 cups)
- Yellow mustard (.5 cups)
- Ketchup (1 cup)
- Apple cider vinegar (1 cup)
- Beef roast (2 lbs.)

Nutrition Information:

Protein: 25 grams

Carbs: 17 grams

Fats: 16.8 grams

Saturated Fats: 1.2 grams

Sugar: 8.7 grams

Fiber .5 grams

Calories: 313

PREPARATION

- Add 1 cup of water as well as the beef to a slow cooker and let them cook, covered, on a low setting for 6 hours.
1. Once the ingredients are done cooking, discard the bones and add everything else to a blender and blend well prior to serving.
2. At the 5 hour mark, start to prepare the barbeque sauce by taking a saucepan and adding gin the cayenne, paprika, garlic powder, onion powder, Worcestershire sauce, hot sauce, brown sugar, yellow mustard, ketchup and apple cider vinegar and mixing well before placing it on top of a burner over a stove set to a high heat.
3. Let the sauce boil 5 minutes, regularly stirring.
4. After the slow cooker, has finished cooking the beef, remove it and drain the slow cooker before adding in the beef as well as 60 percent of the sauce.
5. Cook everything for 30 minutes on a high heat and top with the remaining sauce prior to serving.

DELICIOUS SLOW COOKER STEW

Serving Size: 1

Servings per Recipe: 4

Smart Points per Serving: 7

Calories: 290

Cooking Time: Approx. 6 Hours

Ingredients:

- Beef broth (8 cups)
- Garlic (4 cloves minced)
- Onion (1 large, chopped)
- Carrots (4 medium peeled, chopped)
- Potatoes (4 peeled, chopped)

- Chuck roast (2 lbs. beef, cubed)
- Ground black pepper (as needed)
- Sea salt (to taste)
- Celery (4 stalks chopped)

Nutrition Information:

Protein: 27 grams

Carbs: 20 grams

Fats: 11 grams

Saturated Fats: 3 grams

Sugar: 3 grams

Fiber 3 grams

Calories: 290

PREPARATION

1. Add all of the ingredients, except for the celery to a slow cooker and let them cook, covered, on a high setting for 6 hours.
2. 20 minutes before the stew is done cooking, add in the celery.
3. Serve and enjoy!

WHITE CHEDDAR BROCCOLI MAC & CHEESE:

Serving Size: 1

Servings per Recipe: 4

Smart Points per Serving: 13

Calories: 387

Cooking Time: Approx. 2 Hours

Ingredients:

- 1/2 cups milk
- 2 egg whites
- 2 teaspoons cornstarch or custard starch
- 1/8 teaspoon nutmeg
- 1 cup ground white cheddar
- 1 little head of broccoli, cut into nibble measured florets
- 2 cups dry, entire wheat pasta

Nutrition Information:

Saturated Fat: 7g

Cholesterol: 38mg

Sodium: 285mg

Carbohydrates: 48g

Sugar: 7g

Protein: 21g

PREPARATION

1. Whisk together the milk, egg whites and cornstarch in the cooker embeds. Make certain to whisk well.
2. Blend in the ground cheddar, broccoli and pasta shells.
3. Cook on low for 1-1/2 to 2 hours.
4. After the main hour, mix the sustenance on a semi-consistent premise.
5. This will do two things. It will permit the pasta to cook equally.

6.   It will likewise permit you to watch out for the pasta and see when it's set.

7.   Each moderate cooker is distinctive, so the planning for this formula might be marginally unique on this for you.

8.   Pasta goes from "cooked" to "mush" rapidly.

9.   So make certain to continue mixing every so often to watch out for things.

SLOW COOKER TACOS

Serving Size: 2
Servings per Recipe: 8
Smart Points per Serving: 8
Calories: 288
Cooking Time: Approx. 6 Hours

Ingredients:
- 6 inch tortillas (8)
- Bay leaves (2)
- Ground black pepper (to taste)
- Thyme (.25 tsp. dried)
- Cilantro (1 cup chopped)
- Cayenne pepper (.25 tsp.)
- Cinnamon (.5 tsp.)
- Cumin (.5 tsp. ground)
- Chuck roast (2 lbs. beef, cubed)
- Garlic (8 cloves minced)
- Onion (1 chopped)
- Tomatoes (2 chopped)
- 2 jalapeno peppers (chopped, seeded)
- Oil (1 T)

Nutrition Information:
Protein: 19 grams
Carbs: 15 grams
Fats: 17 grams
Saturated Fats: 2.1 gram
Sugar: .5 grams
Fiber 2 grams
Calories: 288

PREPARATION

1.   Add the oil to a skillet and place it on the stove over a burner set to a medium/high heat.

2.   Add in the garlic as well as the onion, tomatoes and peppers and let them cook for 5 minutes before removing them from the pan and adding them to a blender with 1 tsp. salt and .5 cups water and blend well.

3.   Add the results back into the skillet before mixing in the beef and turning the burner to medium and let it brown.

4.   Mix in the cayenne pepper, cinnamon and cumin and let everything cook for an additional minute.

5.   As this cooks, add 1.5 cups of water as well as the thyme and cilantro into the blender and blend well.

6.   Add all of the ingredients to the slow cooker and let them cook, covered, on a low heat for 6 hours.

7.   Discard the bay leaves prior to adding the ingredients to the tortillas and serving.

MUSHROOMS BEEF TIPS OVER NOODLES

Serving Size: 1
Servings per Recipe: 4
Smart Points per Serving: 10
Calories: 364
Cooking Time: Approx. 6 Hours

Ingredients:

- Egg noodles (2 cups cooked)
- Water (.25 cups cold)
- Cornstarch (2 T)
- Worcestershire sauce (1 T)
- Beef broth (2 cups)
- Red wine (.3 cups)
- Olive oil (2 tsp.)
- Salt (.5 tsp.)
- Beef tips (1 lb.)
- Onion (1 sliced, halved)
- Mushrooms (.5 lbs.)

Nutrition Information:

Protein: 29 grams
Carbs: 29 grams
Fats: 11.8 grams
Saturated Fats: 6.9 grams
Sugar: 2 grams
Fiber 1 grams
Calories: 364

PREPARATION

1.   Place the onion and the mushrooms into the slow cooker.

2.   Season the meet as needed before placing it, along with the oil, into a skillet before placing the skillet onto the stove on top of a burner set to a high/medium heat.

3.   Let the meat brown before adding it into the slow cooker.

4.   Ensure the skillet is deglazed before adding in the Worcestershire sauce as well as the broth and mixing well.

5.   Add the results to the slower cooker and let everything cook on a low heat for 6 hours.

6.   Combine the water and cornstarch, add the results to the slow cooker and let everything cook on high for 15 minutes.

7.   Plate the noodles and top with the beef tip mixture prior to serving.

ONE POT BEEF RAGU

Serving Size: 1
Servings per Recipe: 10
Smart Points per Serving: 5
Calories: 224
Cooking Time: Approx. 8 Hours
Ingredients:
- Thyme (2 T chopped)
- Rosemary (2 T chopped)
- Bay leaves (2)
- Beef broth (1.5 cups)
- Tomatoes (14.5 oz. crushed)
- Tomatoes (14.5 oz. diced)
- Garlic (4 cloves minced)
- Carrot (1 diced)
- Onion (.5 diced)
- Celery (1 rib diced)
- Lean been (2.5 lbs.)

Nutrition Information:
Protein: 29 grams
Carbs: 6 grams
Fats: 9 grams
Saturated Fats: 4 grams
Sugar: 3 grams
Fiber 2 grams
Calories: 224

PREPARATION
1.   Add all of the ingredients to the slow cooker before covering it, setting it to a low temperature and letting it cook for eight hours.

SLOW COOK BEEF LASAGNA

Serving Size: 2
Servings per Recipe: 6
Smart Points per Serving: 11
Calories: 360
Cooking Time: Approx. 6 Hours
Ingredients:
- Parmesan cheese (.5 cups shredded)
- Lasagna noodles (6)
- Mozzarella cheese (1.5 cups shredded)
- Ricotta cheese (1 cup)
- Red pepper flakes (.25 tsp.)
- Basil (.5 tsp. dried)
- Oregano (1 tsp. dried)
- Salt (1 tsp.)

- Tomato sauce (15 oz.)
- Tomato (28 oz. crushed)
- Garlic (1 clove minced)
- Onion (1 chopped)
- Ground beef (1 lb.)

Nutrition Information:

Protein: 28 grams

Carbs: 31 grams

Fats: 14 grams

Saturated Fats: 7 grams

Sugar: 2 grams

Fiber 1 grams

Calories: 360

PREPARATION

1. Place a skillet on the stove on top of a burner set to a high/medium heat before adding in the garlic, onion and beef and letting the beef brown.
2. Add in the red pepper flakes, basil, oregano, salt, tomato sauce and crushed tomatoes and let the results simmer 5 minutes.
3. Combine the mozzarella and the ricotta cheese.
4. Add .3 of the total sauce from the skillet and add it to the slow cooker. Place 3 noodles on top of the sauce, followed by cheese mixture. Create three layers total.
5. Cover the slow cooker and let it cook on a low heat for 6 hours.

DELICIOUS MEXICAN MEATLOAF:

Serving Size: 1-inch thick slice

Servings per Recipe: 6

Smart Points per Serving: 9

Calories: 335

Cooking Time: Approx. 6 Hours

Ingredients:

For Meatloaf:

- 2 tablespoons olive oil
- 1 onion, slashed
- 1 jalapeño, minced
- 1 clove garlic, minced
- 1 pound ground hamburger
- 1 teaspoon ground cumin
- 1/4 teaspoon cayenne pepper
- 1/2 teaspoon ocean salt
- 1/4 teaspoon dark pepper
- 1/2 cup moved oats, coarsely ground in a sustenance processor
- 1 egg

For Coat:

- 1 cup diced tomatoes in juice
- 1 clove garlic, minced

- 1 tablespoon nectar
- 1 tablespoon lime juice
- 1 canned chipotle stew in adobo sauce
- 1/4 teaspoon Kosher salt

Nutrition Information:

Saturated Fat: 3 g

Cholesterol: 111mg

Sodium: 534 mg

Carbohydrates: 12 g

Sugars: 5 g

Protein: 30 g

PREPARATION

1. Warm a skillet over medium warmth. Include the olive oil, onions, and jalapeño.
2. Cook until delicate and include the garlic. Cook for 1 moment and add to a huge bowl.
3. Blend in the hamburger and seasonings and blend well. At the point when the blend is marginally cool, include the oats and egg.
4. Shape the blend into a round chunk and exchange to a moderate cooker pot. Cover and cook on low, for 6 hours.
5. Before serving, make the coating by consolidating the greater part of the fixings in a little pan. Heat until it starts boiling.
6. Cook for 5 minutes and exchange to a blender. Mix until smooth.
7. Spoon the meatloaf before serving.

ASIAN TASTE CHICKEN CURRY:

Serving Size: 1 cup

Servings per Recipe: 6

Smart Points per Serving: 11

Calories: 309

Cooking Time: Approx. 4 Hours

Ingredients:

- 1 pound boneless skinless chicken, cut into bite-size pieces
- 1 medium onion daintily cut
- 1 (15 ounces) can chickpeas
- 4-6 little red potatoes, cubed
- 4 medium carrots, chopped
- 1/2 cups coconut milk
- 1/2 cup chicken stock
- 3-4 extensive tomatoes, cleaved
- 2 tablespoons tomato puree
- 2 tablespoons curry powder
- 2 teaspoons salt
- 1/2 teaspoon cayenne pepper
- 1/2 teaspoon ground cumin
- 1 cup green peas, solidified
- 2 tablespoons lemon juice

- 1 teaspoon new ground ginger
- 1/4 cup chopped cilantro, discretionary

Nutrition Information:

Saturated Fat: 8 g

Cholesterol: 0 mg

Sodium: 543 mg

Carbohydrates: 39 g

Sugars: 6 g

Protein: 18 g

PREPARATION

1. Least moderate cooker estimate: 5 Quarts
2. Combine coconut milk, chicken stock, tomato puree, curry powder, salt, cumin, and cayenne.
3. Include chicken bosoms, onion, chickpeas, carrots, tomatoes, and potatoes. Cook on high for 4 hours.
4. Include solidified peas, lemon juice, and crisp ginger amid the most recent 10 minutes of cooking.
5. On the other hand, on the off chance that you don't plan to serve immediately include these last ingredients while the ease back cooker is set to warm.

SLOW COOK BEEF CHILI

Serving Size: 1

Servings per Recipe: 12

Smart Points per Serving: 4

Calories: 138

Cooking Time: Approx. 5 Hours

Ingredients:

- Ground black pepper (to taste)
- Sea salt (to taste)
- Tomato paste (2 T)
- Green chilies (.25 cups diced)
- Sweet onion (1 chopped)
- Kidney beans (15 oz. rinsed, drained)
- Tomatoes (28 oz. crushed)
- Cumin (2 tsp.)
- Chili powder (2 T)
- Green bell pepper (1 diced, seeded)
- Red bell pepper (1 diced, seeded)
- Garlic (1 T minced)
- Ground beef (1 lb.)

Nutrition Information:

Protein: 13 grams

Carbs: 17 grams

Fats: 3 grams

Saturated Fats: 1 grams

Sugar: 2 grams
Fiber 5 grams
Calories: 138

PREPARATION

1.   Place a skillet on the stove on top of a burner set to a high/medium heat before adding in the garlic, onion and beef and letting the beef brown.

2.   Drain the fat from the pan and return the meet to it before adding in the bell peppers and cooking for 5 minutes prior to seasoning using the cumin and chili powder.

3.   Add the tomato paste, green chilies, onion, kidney beans, tomatoes and meat mix into the slow cooker and mix well. Cook on high, covered for 5 hours.

4.   Season to taste prior to serving.

CHICKEN WITH MUSHROOM GRAVY:

Serving Size: 1
Servings per Recipe: 4
Smart Points per Serving: 10
Calories: 341
Cooking Time: Approx. 4 Hours

Ingredients:

- 1 tablespoon additional virgin olive oil
- 4 cuts without nitrate bacon, diced (we utilized turkey bacon)
- 4 boneless, skinless lean chicken bosom filets
- 16 ounces cut cremini mushrooms
- 1 yellow onion daintily cut into rings
- 2 cloves garlic, minced
- 1/2 teaspoon dark pepper
- 1 teaspoon legitimate or ocean salt
- 1/4 cup new level leaf parsley, slashed
- 1/2 cups chicken soup, low-sodium, sans fat
- 2 tablespoons flour

Nutrition Information:

Saturated Fat: 5g
Cholesterol: 81mg
Sodium: 874mg
Carbohydrates: 15g
Sugar: 5g
Protein: 28g

PREPARATION

1.   Add oil to an extensive skillet, swing to medium-high warmth, include diced bacon and cook until fresh.

2.   Exchange to a plate with a paper towel on it. Add chicken to the skillet and burn chicken on both sides just until brilliant cocoa.

3.   Remove and put on a paper towel.

4.   Diminish warmth to medium-low, add onion to a similar skillet, and sauté until delicate, around 4 minutes.

5.   Add chicken to a moderate cooker, and then cover with diced bacon, onion, and remaining ingredients, aside from the flour.

6.   Wrap and roast on low temperature for 3 to 4 hours, or on high temperature for 1 to 3 hours, or until the chicken is done and effectively drops with a fork.

7.   Expel chicken from moderate cooker and put aside. Add flour to a moderate cooker and race until smooth.

8.   Return chicken to moderate cooker and keep cooking until sauce is thick 10-15 minutes.

9.   When you add the onion to the skillet, pour in around a 1/4 cup soup to deglaze the dish and get every one of the bits on the base of the container from the chicken and afterward add to the moderate cooker.

ITALIAN CHICKEN AND SWEET POTATOES:

Serving Size: 1 ½ cups
Servings per Recipe: 4
Smart Points per Serving: 10
Calories: 364
Cooking Time: Approx. 4 Hours

Ingredients:
*   4 boneless skinless chicken breasts,
*   8 ounces cremini mushrooms sliced
*   2 cups diced sweet potatoes
*   1/4 cup new lemon juice
*   1/2 cup chicken stock
*   1/4 cup olive oil
*   1 teaspoon dried oregano
*   1 teaspoon dried parsley
*   1 teaspoon dried basil
*   1 teaspoon genuine or ocean salt
*   1/2 teaspoon black pepper
*   1/2 teaspoon onion powder
*   2 garlic cloves, minced

Nutrition Information:
Saturated Fat: 2g
Cholesterol: 62mg
Sodium: 700mg
Carbohydrates: 33g
Sugar: 8g
Protein: 24g

PREPARATION
1.   Put the chicken in center of the moderate cooker, and after that put the sweet potatoes on the opposite side of the mushrooms.

2.   In another bowl, whisk the rest of the fixings together, then pour over the fixings in the moderate cooker.

3.   Cover up and cook on low temperature for 6 to 7 hours or on high flame for 3to 4 hours.

DELICIOUS TAMARI GLAZED CHICKEN:

Serving Size: 1
Servings per Recipe: 8
Smart Points per Serving: 5
Calories: 176
Cooking Time: Approx. 6 to 8 Hours

Ingredients:

- 8 boneless chicken thighs, skin removed
- 1 tablespoon Chinese 5-flavor powder
- 1 tablespoon olive oil
- 2 white onions, generally cleaved
- 1 cup low-sodium chicken stock
- 1/3 cup rice vinegar
- 1/3 cup tamari
- 1 tablespoon coconut sugar
- 1 teaspoon red bean stew pieces
- 1 bay leaf
- 1/2 cup pea pods
- 2 scallions cut

Nutrition Information:

Saturated Fat: 3g
Cholesterol: 43mg
Sodium: 714mg
Carbohydrates: 7g
Sugar: 3g
Protein: 14g

PREPARATION

1. Season the chicken thighs with the Chinese 5-flavor powder.
2. Warm the oil in a substantial skillet over medium-high warmth.
3. Include the chicken and cook until caramelized on both sides, 3-4 minutes.
4. Lay the onions in the base of your moderate cooker pot, and lay the chicken pieces on top.
5. Whisk the juices, vinegar, tamari, coconut sugar, red stew pieces, and bay leaf together and pour over the chicken.
6. Cover up and cook on low temperature for 6 to 8 hours or on high flame for 3 to 4 hours.
7. At the point when the chicken is done, include the pea pods and cook 10 minutes, or until delicate.
8. Serve with the scallions.

BROWN RICE AND CHICKEN:

Serving Size: 1 cup
Servings per Recipe: 8
Smart Points per Serving: 7
Calories: 289
Cooking Time: Approx. 6 Hours

Ingredients:

For the Rice:
- 2 cups natural Brown Rice
- 5 cups water
- 1 14.5oz. can natural prepared cut diced tomatoes (don't drain)
- 4 ribs natural celery, flushed and diced
- ½ substantial sweet white onion, slashed
- Siracha hot bean stew sauce
- Natural herb blend (no salt) approx. 2 tablespoon
- ½ to 1 teaspoon cumin
- ½ teaspoon paprika

For the Chicken:
- 4 natural boneless/skinless chicken breasts
- ¼ to ½ cup gourmet Yoshida sauce
- Siracha hot bean stew sauce (squirt to cover the highest point of the chicken)
- Substantial sprinkling of natural herb blend (no salt)
- 1 tablespoon pounded red bean stew peppers
- 1 teaspoon cumin
- 1 teaspoon paprika
- ½ teaspoon cayenne pepper (discretionary)
- 2 crisp rosemary sprigs

Nutrition Information:

Saturated Fat: 0.8 g

Cholesterol: 44 mg

Sodium: 53 mg

Carbohydrates: 40.5 g

Sugars: 2.1 g

Protein: 20.8 g

TURKEY LASAGNA SOUP:

Serving Size: 1 cup

Servings per Recipe: 8

Smart Points per Serving: 9

Calories: 314

Cooking Time: Approx. 6 to 8 Hours

Ingredients:
- 1 pound lean ground turkey
- 1 (24 ounces) bump tomato basil marinara, no sugar included
- 4 cups chicken juices, low-sodium
- 8 sprigs new (wavy or level) parsley
- 1/2 teaspoon legitimate or ocean salt
- 1/2 teaspoon black pepper
- 8 entire wheat lasagna noodles, broken into fourths
- 1 cup (part-skim) mozzarella cheddar
- 1/2 cup ricotta cheddar, decreased fat

- New basil for trimming, discretionary

Nutrition Information:

Saturated Fat: 5g

Cholesterol: 66mg

Sodium: 336

Carbohydrates: 28g

Sugars: 3g

Protein: 25g

PREPARATION

1. In a skillet over medium warmth, cook ground turkey, parting ways with a fork.
2. Cook only until there's no pink. Deplete off any fat.
3. Add to the moderate cooker, cooked ground turkey, marinara, chicken juices, parsley sprigs, salt, and pepper.
4. Cover and cook on low 4-6 hours. The most recent 30 minutes of cooking time, include broken lasagna noodles, mozzarella.
5. Check noodles to ensure they are delicate, however not soft. Evacuate parsley sprigs before serving, if fancied.
6. Serve in dishes with a touch of ricotta cheddar and trimming with crisp basil, if fancied.

BEEF BOURGUIGNON STEW:

Serving Size: 1 cup

Servings per Recipe: 8

Smart Points per Serving: 8

Calories: 310

Cooking Time: Approx. 6 Hours

Ingredients:

- 1/2 pounds lean hamburger hurl, cut into chomp measure solid shapes
- 1 pound reddish brown (Idaho) potatoes, peeled and cleaved into extensive blocks
- 2 carrots, cleaved into 1/2 inch thick cuts
- 2 stalks celery thickly cut
- 3 tablespoons additional virgin olive oil, partitioned
- 1 entire sprig rosemary
- 1 teaspoon dry oregano
- 1 pound white catch mushrooms, divided
- 3 thyme sprigs
- 1 bay leaf
- 2 cloves garlic, minced
- 3 tablespoons white entire wheat flour or universally handy flour
- 1 cup low-sodium hamburger stock
- 3 cups pinot noir
- 10 pearl onions, divided or 1 medium yellow or white onion, diced
- 1 teaspoon fit or sea salt
- 1/2 teaspoon black pepper

Nutrition Information:

Saturated Fat: 2g

Cholesterol: 54mg
Sodium: 141mg
Carbohydrates: 19g
Sugars: 3g
Protein: 23g
PREPARATION
1.   Sprinkle hamburger 3D squares with 1/2 teaspoon salt and 1/2 teaspoon pepper. Dig in flour to coat.
2.   Put 1/2 tablespoon of olive oil in the skillet over medium-high warmth.
3.   Include a large portion of the meat 3D shapes and chestnut on all sides, for around 5 minutes.
4.   It is not important to cook the hamburger completely through, simply burn the exterior.
5.   Rehash with the second bunch. Put the hamburger aside.
6.   In a similar container that the hamburger was cooked in, include 1/4 cup of the wine and rub the base, permitting a portion of the fluid to vanish.
7.   Include herbs, mushrooms, pearl onions or diced onion, celery, carrots, and 1 more tablespoon of olive oil and cook for around 5 minutes.
8.   Include garlic and cook for an extra 30 seconds.
9.   Empty everything from the dish into the moderate cooker. Include whatever is left of the wine, the stock, whatever is left of the salt, the bay leaf, the potatoes, and meat solid shapes.
10.   Cover up and cook on low temperature for 6 to 8 hours or on high flame for 3 to 4 hours.

SLOW COOK FIESTA CHILI SUPPER:

Serving Size: 1 cup
Servings per Recipe: 6
Smart Points per Serving: 7
Calories: 254
Cooking Time: Approx. 6 Hours
Ingredients:
*   1 pound lean ground turkey
*   1 (15 ounces) can red kidney beans, depleted and flushed
*   1 clove garlic, minced
*   1/2 cup slashed onion
*   3 cups low sodium chicken or vegetable juices
*   1/2 cups solidified corn bits
*   1/2 cup diced red ringer pepper
*   2 tablespoons bean stew powder, in addition to additional to taste
*   1 teaspoon cumin
*   1 chipotle chili (from can), minced with seeds, in addition to 2 tablespoons sauce from can
*   1 lime, cut into wedges, for serving
*   1/2 teaspoon fit or ocean salt
*   1/2 teaspoon black pepper
Nutrition Information:
Saturated Fat: 2g
Cholesterol: 56mg

Sodium: 459mg
Carbohydrates: 24g
Sugar: 5g
Protein: 22g
PREPARATION
1. In a medium skillet cook ground turkey just until it loses its pink shading.
2. Get rid of any fat and add to the moderate cooker.
3. Add every single outstanding fixing to the moderate cooker and cook on low for 6 to 8 hours.
4. Present with lime wedges to crush into a stew, if needed.
5. Discretionary fixing thoughts incorporate nonfat sharp cream or Greek yogurt, cleaved cilantro, or scallions.

VEGETARIAN ENCHILADAS:

Serving Size: 3
Servings per Recipe: 12
Smart Points per Serving: 13
Calories: 464
Cooking Time: Approx. 4 to 6 Hours
Ingredients:
For Sauce:
- 2 tablespoons olive oil
- 2 tablespoons flour
- 1/4 cup bean stew powder
- 1/2 teaspoon garlic powder
- 1/2 teaspoon salt
- 1/4 teaspoon ground cumin
- 1/4 teaspoon Mexican oregano
- 2 cups vegetable stock

For Enchiladas:
- 1 tablespoon olive oil
- 1 onion, diced
- 1 cup cooked dark beans
- 1/4 cup cleaved new cilantro
- Juice of 1 lime
- 12 corn tortillas
- 1 cup lessened fat destroyed cheddar, separated down the middle
- Lessened fat sharp cream and new hacked cilantro, for serving

Nutrition Information:
Saturated Fat: 2 g
Cholesterol: 0mg
Sodium: 405 mg
Carbohydrates: 72 g
Sugars: 3 g
Protein: 16 g

PREPARATION

1.   Make the sauce by warming a medium pan over medium warmth. Include the olive oil and flour and mix until smooth and bubbly.

2.   Include the seasonings and mix until all around joined. Add the stock and heat to the point of boiling.

3.   Lessen warmth and stew for 5 minutes.

4.   Make the enchilada filling by warming a huge skillet over medium-high warmth. Include the olive oil, trailed by the onions.

5.   Cook until the onions are delicate, season with salt and pepper, and include the beans.

6.   Cook for around 2 minutes and include the cilantro and lime juice. Kill warm.

7.   To make the enchiladas, put the corn tortillas on a plate and cover with a moist paper towel.

8.   Microwave for 1 minute, or until tortillas are delicate and malleable.

9.   Fill every tortilla with around 2 tablespoons of filling and top with a sprinkling of cheddar.

10.   Move up and lay in your moderate cooker, pressing them in firmly so they remain together.

11.   On the off chance that the tortillas cool, you may need to warm them.

12.   When the greater part of the enchiladas is in the cooker, pour the sauce over top of them, ensuring they are very much secured.

13.   Cover and cook on low warmth for 4-6 hours. Before serving, sprinkle remaining cheddar on top, cover, and cook on low for 15 minutes, or until cheddar is liquefied.

14.   Present with sharp cream and new cleaved cilantro.

JAMBALAYA WITH CHICKEN AND SHRIMP:

Serving Size: 1 ½ cups
Servings per Recipe: 4
Smart Points per Serving: 12
Calories: 465
Cooking Time: Approx. 8 Hours

Ingredients:

- 1 pound chicken breasts, cut into bite estimated pieces
- 1 onion, diced
- 1 green pepper, diced
- 4 stalks celery, diced
- 1 cup custom made chicken stock
- 1 tablespoons dried oregano
- 1 tablespoons Cajun or Creole flavoring
- 1 teaspoon hot sauce, or more to taste
- 1 teaspoon dried thyme
- 1 bay leaf
- 1 (28 ounces) can diced tomatoes
- 1 pound peeled and deveined shrimp, tails removed
- 2 cups cooked chestnut rice
- Kosher salt and new ground black pepper, to taste

- New cleaved parsley, for embellishment

Nutrition Information:

Saturated Fat: 3 g

Cholesterol: 101

Sodium: 1125 mg

Carbohydrates: 50 g

Sugars: 8 g

Protein: 40 g

PREPARATION

1. Consolidate everything aside from the shrimp, rice, and parsley in the moderate cooker.
2. Cook over low warmth for 8 hours.
3. Add the shrimp into the pan, fry for 20 minutes in anticipation of suitable for eating.
4. Serve over the rice with newly slashed parsley on top.

SLOW COOK LASAGNA TURKEY:

Serving Size: 1 slice

Servings per Recipe: 8

Smart Points per Serving: 6

Calories: 199

Cooking Time: Approx. 6 Hours

Ingredients:

- 1 pound lean ground turkey, or lean ground hamburger
- 1 vast onion, diced
- 3 cloves garlic, minced
- 2 (25 ounces) cups pasta sauce, no sugar included
- 2 cups low-fat curds
- 8 ounces destroyed (part skim) mozzarella cheddar
- 1 teaspoon Italian flavoring
- Squeeze of salt
- 12 (uncooked) entire wheat lasagna noodles, (soften up half before adding to moderate cooker)
- 1/2 cup naturally ground Parmesan cheddar
- Crisp basil, for enhancement

Nutrition Information:

Saturated Fat: 5 g

Cholesterol: 78

Sodium: 1015 mg

Carbohydrates: 33 g

Sugars: 8 g

Protein: 38 g

PREPARATION

1. Add the turkey and onion to a huge skillet and cook over medium warmth until the turkey has lost its pink shading.
2. Include the garlic and cook for one extra moment. Empty any fat out of the cooked turkey.
3. Include 1/2 cup pasta sauce and mix to join.

4.   Join the curds, mozzarella, Italian flavoring, and salt.
5.   Include a 1/2 cup meat sauce to the base of the moderate cooker. Next, include a layer of lasagna noodles and spread 1/4 cheddar blend over noodles.
6.   Rehash the layers until these fixings are no more.
7.   Cover and cook in the moderate cooker on low warmth until noodles are still somewhat firm and cheddar is bubbly roughly 4-6 hours.
8.   Evacuate the top and add the parmesan to the top. Kill the moderate cooker and permit the goulash to sit for 15 minutes before cutting.
9.   In the event that coveted, serve decorated with the crisp basil and extra parmesan.

DELICIOUS HOISIN CHICKEN

Prep time: 10 mins
Cook time: 1 ½ hours
Servings: 4 cups of this
Points: 4

Ingredients:
- ½ cup low-sodium soy sauce
- ½ cup low sodium chicken broth
- 2 T of minced ginger and agave nectar or honey
- ½ t of chili garlic sauce, more to taste
- 1 T cornstarch
- Sliced onions for garnish
- ½ cup hoisin sauce
- 2 pounds of boneless, skinless chicken thighs, with the fat cut off
- 2 T water

PREPARATION
1.   Get a bowl and put in the soy sauce, broth, honey, chili garlic sauce, and ginger
2.   Put the chicken thighs into the slow cooker and the sauce over this
3.   Cook it on high for at least 1 ½ hours, more if you want it tender. If you want it low, do it for about 4 hours
4.   Transfer the chicken and shred t on a cutting board
5.   Pour the sauce into a saucepan and then put together the cornstarch and water, putting it into the sauce
6.   Boil it and let it cook until it's thickened
7.   Put the shredded chicken in a bowl to keep warm and then put about ¾ cup of the sauce over the top of it. You can use the rest for any stir-fried veggies or rice. Coat it and garnish with green onions to serve.

CROCK POT CHICKEN CHILI

Prep time: 10 mins
Cook time: 480 mins
Servings: 8
Points: 5

Ingredients:
- 12 oz. of boneless, skinless chicken breasts, diced together

- 1 quart canned tomatoes
- 1 can of drained kidney beans
- 1 chopped onion
- 1 envelope of chili seasoning mix
- 1 can of undrained corn
- 1 chopped green bell pepper
- ½ cup salsa

PREPARATION

1.	Coat a skillet with cooking spray and sear your chicken
2.	Put the chicken, the seasoning, the tomatoes and corn, the rest of the veggies, and the salsa to your crock pot
3.	Put it on low for 6-8 hours until tender.

GREATEST BUFFALO CHICKEN

Prep time: 10 mins
Cook time: 7-9 hours
Servings: 12 ½ cup servings
Points: 3 per serving

Ingredients:

- 3 pounds of raw, boneless and skinless chicken breasts. You can use it frozen or unfrozen
- 1 oz., packet of dry ranch mix
- 12 oz., bottle of buffalo wing sauce
- 2 T light butter

PREPARATION

1.	Take the chicken and put it in the slow cooker. Put the wing sauce on top of it and ten put the ranch mix on top
2.	Close the lid and cook for about 7-9 hours
3.	You can then shred the meat and from there put it in the sauce and add the butter.
4.	You should cook it once again on low to get the sauce to soak it up. Serve it how you want.
5.	Do take into consideration that if you serve it with a bun, there are more points to be calculated, this is just the chicken alone.

SLOW COOKER LASAGNA

Prep time: 20 mins
Cook time: about 6 hours
Serving size: 6 people
Points: 10

Ingredients:

- 1 pound of uncooked lean ground beef
- 1 minced garlic clove
- 1 can tomato sauce
- 1 t dried oregano and basil
- 1 cup ricotta cheese

- 1 small uncooked and chopped onion
- 28 oz., can have crushed tomatoes
- 1 t table salt
- 1 t crushed red pepper flakes, more to taste
- 2 cups shredded mozzarella cheese, divided
- ½ cup shredded parmesan cheese, one with a strong flavor
- 6 item uncooked lasagna noodles

PREPARATION

1. Heat a skillet and add in the garlic, beef and onion, stirring and cooking it for 5-7 minutes. Add in the crushed tomatoes tomato sauce, spices, salt, red pepper flakes, and let this simmer for at least 5 minutes
2. While it does, stir in the ricotta with a cup of the mozzarella cheese
3. Put 1/3 of the beef into your slow cooker, and then break up half of the lasagna sheets in half and then put it on top, then the ricotta, and then continue this with the rest of the mixture
4. Cover it and let it cook for 4-6 hours
5. Take it off and season to taste if needed
6. When ready, combine the rest of the cheese and put it over the beef mixture. Let it sit in there and wait until the cheese melts and firms up. Spoon about 1/6 of the dish into a plate for the serving size

SLOW COOKER VEGGIE CHILI

Prep time: 20 mins
Cook time: 5 hours
Points: 3 per serving
Serving per recipe: 12

Ingredients:
- 1 pound of lean ground beef or turkey
- 1 large green and 1 large red bell pepper, both seeded and diced
- 2 T chili powder
- 1 can crushed tomatoes
- 1 chopped sweet onion
- 2 T tomato paste
- 1 T minced fresh garlic
- 2 t cumin
- 1 can kidney beans, drained and rinsed
- ½ cup diced green chilles
- Black pepper for taste

PREPARATION

1. Cook the ground beef or your turkey with the garlic in a skillet, using it to pull apart the meat until it is browned
2. Take off any fat and then add in the bell peppers until they are soft, usually about 5 minutes. Add in the chili powder and the cumin
3. Put the ingredients into a slow cooker and then let it sit for about 4-5 hours. You can season to taste with black pepper.

CHEESEBURGER SOUP

Prep time: 15 mins
Cook time: 2 hours
Points: 7
Servings: 8

Ingredients:

- 1 clove of minced garlic
- 1 stalk of chopped celery
- 2 T all-purpose flour
- 1 cup low-fat evaporated milk
- ½ t paprika
- 1/8 t black pepper
- Cooking spray
- 1 chopped onion
- 1 pound uncooked lean ground beef
- 3 cups of canned chicken broth, divided up
- ½ pound cubed reduced fat Velveeta cheese
- ¼ t salt
- 24 crumbled tortilla chips

PREPARATION

1.   Coat a skillet with oil and heat it for about half a minute, putting the garlic, celery, and the onion in there until tender
2.   Coat a slow cooker with cooking spray and put in the veggies, and while doing that, let the beef brown in the same skillet for about five minutes, putting it into a slow cooker
3.   Combine the flour and half of the broth, stirring until lumps are gone
4.   Put the flour broth in the skillet and leave the rest to the side.
5.   Simmer it and scrape anything that's left with a spoon, putting it into the slow cooker. Put the rest of the ingredients in there, and let it sit for about 2 hours
6.   Serve with tortilla chips on top, and as of note, if it cooks for too long, it could separate the cheese so be mindful of this.

ITALIAN PASTA FAGGIOLI

Prep time: 30 mins
Cook time: 7 hours
Servings: 10
Points: 5

Ingredients:

- 1 pound of extra lean ground beef, already browned and drained
- 1 cup of chopped onions and carrots
- 1 can of kidney beans, drained
- 4 cups beef broth of choice
- 1 t oregano
- ½ t salt and black pepper
- ½ cup chopped celery
- 1 can diced tomatoes with the juice intact

- 1 can white beans, drained
- 1 jar of pasta sauce of choice
- 1 t hot pepper sauce
- 2 cups dry pasta
- Grated parmesan for serving
- ¼ cup parsley for serving

PREPARATION
1. Put everything into a slow cooker and mix it together except for pasta
2. Let it cook on low for 5-7 hours or until it's tenderized
3. Put the pasta into the soup and adjust with the spices if desired
4. Serve with parmesan and the parsley if you want it.

SLOW COOKER SWEET AND SOUR CHICKEN

Prep time: 10 mins
Cook time: 420 mins
Servings: 4
Points: 7

Ingredients:
- 2 pound of boneless, skinless chicken breasts
- ¼ t garlic and onion powder
- 1 T brown sugar
- 5 oz., of sweet and sour sauce
- ½ pound pineapple chunks with ¼ of the juice left
- 1 pound frozen stir fry veggies

PREPARATION
1. Cut the chicken and put in all of the ingredients but the veggies
2. Cook this on low for about 6-7 hours
3. Add in the veggies during the last 30 mins of cooking and put it on high heat.

SUGARY PORK TENDERLOIN

Prep time: 5 mins
Cook time: 8 hours
Servings: 6
Points: 6

Ingredients:
- 2 pounds of pork tenderloin
- ½ cup low sodium chicken broth
- 3 T born sugar
- ½ t garlic powder and cumin
- Salt and pepper for taste
- ¼ cup balsamic vinegar
- 2 T soy sauce
- ¼ t chili powder

PREPARATION
1. Put the vinegar, soy sauce, and the both together

2.   Put in the rest of the ingredients, being careful with the salt. Remember, if you want to add more to it, you can after you cook

3.   Rub the pork with the brown sugar and put it in the slow cooker, and then put the vinegar mixture over it

4.   Cook until very tender, usually about 6-8 hours

5.   If you want, you can reduce the cooking liquid to create a nice glaze

6.   If you want a crisper outside, put it in a broiler for at least 4-5 minutes

CHICKEN POT ROAST

Prep time: 10 mins
Cook time: 4 hours
Servings: 6
Points: 5
Ingredients:
* 1 large chicken that can be roasted
* 2 minced garlic cloves
* 1 t black pepper
* 1 t sea salt
* ¼ cup water
* 2 potatoes, cut into cubes
* 2 t olive oil
* 2 t thyme
* 1 t paprika
* 2 stalks of celery
* 1 cup baby carrots

PREPARATION

1.   rinse and dry the chicken, putting some olive oil on top

2.   Mix the spices and put it on the outside of the chicken, putting the garlic in the cavity with some salt and pepper

3.   Put the water into the slow cooker, then the celery, and then the chicken on top with the breast side up which will help prevent the bottom from being too browned

4.   Put some carrots and potatoes in there around chicken

5.   Cook for about 6 hours on low or 4 on high until the chicken is very tender. You can check this with a meat thermometer

6.   You can broil it in a roasting pan until it is browned to how you want it to be. You can garnish with thyme if you so want.

SLOW COOKER TOMATO SOUP

Prep time: 5 mins
Cook time: 600 mins
Servings: 8
Points: 2 per serving
Ingredients:
* 10 oz., of washed baby spinach
* 2 stalks of celery and carrots, chopped up

- 1 minced clove of garlic
- 1 can of diced tomatoes
- 1 T dried basil
- ½ t crushed red pepper flakes
- 1 chopped onion
- 4 cups of low sodium broths
- 2 bay leaves
- 1 t dried oregano

PREPARATION

1. Take all of the ingredients and put them in a slow cooker
2. Cook this on high for 5 hours or low for 8-10, depending on how tender you want this to be.

ADOBO PORK CARNITAS

Prep time: 15 mins
Cook time: 8 hours
Servings: 11
Points: 4

Ingredients:

- 3 pounds of trimmed, boneless shoulder blade roast
- Black pepper for taste
- 2 t cumin
- ¼ t dry oregano
- 2-3 chipotle peppers in adobo sauce, more to taste
- ¼ t dry adobo seasoning
- 2 t salt
- 6 cloves of garlic, slivered
- ½ t sazon
- 1 cup reduced sodium chicken broth
- 2 bay leaves

PREPARATION

1. Season the pork and sauté it on medium high heat for about 10 minutes, browning the sides. Let it cool
2. Insert knife into pork and put the garlic slivers in there, pushing it all the way in so you don't' see them. season with the cumin, sazon, adobo, and oregano all over your meat
3. Put it in the slow cooker and put the bay leaves and the peppers in there. Cook it on low for about 8 hours. You can then combine it with the juices that you have and add more seasonings, letting it cook for another 15 minutes if you so desire.

HEALTHY BLACK BEAN GUMBO

Prep time: 5 mins
Cook time: 4 hours
Servings: 8 servings
Points: 5
Ingredients:

- 1 chopped red onion
- 2 cups of various peppers, chopped up
- 1 can diced tomatoes with the juices intact
- ¼ t black pepper and dried thyme
- 6 cups chicken broth of choice
- 1 stalk chopped celery
- 1 can drained and rinsed black beans
- 9 oz., of chicken sauce, cut into small pieces
- 1 cup white rice

PREPARATION

- Put all of the ingredients into a slow cooker, adding in the spices and mixing it well
- Cover and cook on high for about 4 hours, adjusting seasonings to taste.

SLOW COOKER SLOPPY JOES WITH LENTILS

Prep time: 10 mins
Cook time: 5 hours
Servings: 6 servings, 1 sandwich
Points: 11

Ingredients:

- 4 cups water
- 2 cups lentils of choice
- 1 chopped onion
- 1 bell pepper, chopped up
- 2 cloves minced garlic
- 2 T chili powder
- 2 T molasses
- 3 t salt
- 1 can diced tomatoes
- 2 T apple cider vinegar
- 2 t mustard powder
- 4 T sucanat
- 3 t homemade veggie broth powder
- 1 can tomato paste

PREPARATION

1. Take all of the ingredients up to the chili powder and put it in the crock pot for about 3 hours or until your lentils are done
2. Put the rest of the ingredients in there, and you can leave it uncovered to help thicken it. Do this for at least an hour, check it, and then add more time if necessary.

CHEESY SPAGHETTI WITH TURKEY SAUSAGE

Prep time: 15 mins
Cook time: 2 hours
Servings: 8 servings, about 1 ¼ cups
Points: 12 with turkey sausage, 10 without

Ingredients:

- 1 pound of lean ground turkey sausage
- 1 jar of spaghetti sauce with no sugar
- 1 cup low-fat cottage cheese
- 1 cup low-fat ricotta cheese
- 1 T chopped fresh basil or a teaspoon of dried basil
- ½ t ground black pepper
- ½ pound of whole week spaghetti, uncooked and broken into small pieces before you add meat
- 1 cup shredded skim mozzarella cheese
- 1 t dried oregano
- Salt to taste

For the turkey sausage:
- 1 pound lean ground turkey or chicken
- ½ t ground black pepper
- 1 t dried oregano
- ½ t garlic powder
- 1 t dried sage
- ½ t cayenne pepper

PREPARATION

1. Put the sausage ingredients and mix it together. Cook it on high and break the pieces until the turkey isn't pink anymore.
2. Take it off the heat and get rid of any fat, combining the meat with the marinara
3. Put the rest of the ingredients together with the turkey, and cook it on low for about 2 hours until the cheese bubbles. You can also add in the spaghetti later, stirring it and then cooking for another hour if desired. If you don't' put in the spaghetti right away, you might have to cook it for another hour or so.

BALSAMIC GLAZED PORK

Prep time: 10 mins
Cook time: 6 hours
Servings: 1 pork chop, 4 servings
Points: 10

Ingredients:
- 2 pounds of thick pork chopped, trimmed of fat
- 2 cups of green beans with the tough ends taken off
- 3 apples, cored and cut into wedges
- 2 heaping cups of chopped carrots
- 1 cup of fat free stock of choice

Marinade:
- 2 T balsamic vinegar
- ¼ t of dried rosemary and oregano
- ½ t dried thyme
- 1 T Dijon mustard
- ¼ cup low sodium soy sauce. You can also use coconut aminos
- 2 cloves of finely chopped garlic

- 2 T of honey
- 1 t ground black pepper

PREPARATION

1. Mix and put the chops in the marinade. Refrigerate it overnight
2. Put the pork chops in a pan and sear it on both sides, usually a couple of minutes on high heat until it's browned
3. Take it out of the pan and get any bits off the bottom with the marinade
4. Put the stock and veggies into the slow cooker, with the meat on top. Cook it for about 4-6 hours, or until they're cooked and tender. Serve immediately.

SLOW COOKER PORTO BEEF

Prep time: 15 mins
Cook time: 6-8 hours
Servings: 4
Points: 9

Ingredients:

- ½ pound Portobello mushrooms
- 1 pound beef steak, cubed
- 2 T olive oil
- 2 cups beef broth
- 2 T cornstarch
- 2 cups cooked egg noodles
- 1 sliced onion
- ½ t salt
- ¼ cup red wine
- 1 T Worcestershire sauce
- ¼ cup cold water

PREPARATION

1. Put the onions and mushrooms into the slow cooker
2. Season the beef to taste with salt and pepper
3. Brown the beef on high in a skillet with oil
4. Put meat in slow cooker and use wine and about 1/3 of the broth that beef was in to deglaze it
5. Put the broth and the Worcestershire sauce together until mixed, adding it to the slow cooker
6. Cook on low for 6-8 hours or until meat becomes tender
7. Put the cornstarch and water together and then put it into the slow cooker for about 15-30 minutes, or until it's reached the right consistency
8. Cook the egg noodles, and then serve the beef tips with the mushroom gravy and the egg noodles for best results.

SLOW COOKER BARBACOA

Prep time: 10 mins
Cook time: 6-8 hours
Servings: 10

Points: 7

Ingredients:

- 3 pounds of chuck roast, cut into chunks
- 1 can diced green chilles
- 6 cloves minced garlic
- 1 T cumin
- 2 t salt
- Juice from 3 different limes
- 1 diced onion
- 2-3 chopped chipotles in adobo sauce
- 2 T apple cider vinegar
- 1 T coriander
- 1 t black pepper
- ½ cup of fat free beef broth of choice

PREPARATION

1. Take all of your ingredients and put them into the slow cooker, mixing them.
2. Cook on low for 6-8 hours or until your meat can be shredded
3. Shred the meat and mix with the juices
4. Serve with a fork for best results

SLOW COOKER BEEF AND CAULIFLOWER MASH

Prep time: 15 mins
Cook time: 8 hours
Servings: 6
Points: 8

Ingredients:

- 2 pounds of cubed beef stew meat
- 5 cloves minced garlic
- 1 cup beef broth
- 1 T smoked paprika
- 2 T light butter
- Salt and pepper for taste
- 1 chopped large onion
- 1 can diced tomatoes with roasted garlic
- 2 T Worcestershire sauce
- 1 head of cauliflower
- ¼ cup sour cream

PREPARATION

1. Mist a skillet with cooking spray and cook on medium high heat. Season your cubes and then brown them in the skillet well. Put them in the crock pot
2. Put the tomatoes, Worcestershire sauce, onions, broth, and garlic into there and mix it with the beef
3. Cook it for about 8-10 hours

4.   Before it's ready to serve, about 15 mins, you should steam the cauliflower until it becomes tender. Drain and put it in a bowl and then mash it with the butter and sour cream together. Season as desired

5.   Serve your beef over the mash and with some mixed greens for best results.

SLOW COOKER ASIAN CHICKEN NOODLES WITH BROCCOLI

Prep time: 10 mins
Cook time: 6 hours
Servings: 6
Points: 7

Ingredients:

- 2 pounds of skinless and boneless chicken breasts
- 1 pound bag of broccoli florets
- ½ cup hoisin sauce
- 3 T rice vinegar
- 1 T minced ginger
- 1 chili pepper to use as a garnish, optional
- 6 oz., of soba noodles, left uncooked
- 3 minced garlic cloves
- 2 T cornstarch
- ¼ cup soy sauce
- 1 t sesame oil

PREPARATION

1.   Mix the hoisin and soy sauces, garlic, cornstarch, ginger, and sesame oil with the water. Make sure it's combined

2.   Add in chicken and then make sure the ingredients are coated. Cook for about 6 hours on low heat

3.   About 30 minutes before it's done, cook the soba noodles, adding the broccoli in the last couple of minutes

4.   Divide into bowls, shredding the chicken and adding the rice vinegar. Put the chicken and sauce over the broccoli and soba noodles. You can serve it with the diced chilles and chili pepper if you desire.

CHICKEN CORDON BLEU

Prep time: 5 mins
Cook time: 3 hours
Servings: 4
Points: 7

Ingredients:

- 4 chicken breasts, boneless and skinless
- ½ cup fat-free milk
- 1 cup bread stuffing mix
- 1 can fat-free condensed cream of chicken soup
- 4 slices lean ham
- ½ cup blue cheese crumbles

PREPARATION

1.   Take the chicken soup and milk and mix it, pour it into the slow cooker to cover bottom
2.   Put the chickens over this
3.   Cover it with the ham, and then ¼ cup of the bleu cheese crumbles
4.   Cover and cook on low for at least 4-6 hours, 2-3 if you choose to use high heat

BACON WITH RANCH DRESSING CHICKEN

Prep time: 15 mins
Cook time: 3.5 hours
Servings: 4
Points: 6

Ingredients:

- 1 pound of boneless, skinless chicken breasts
- 3 cups plain, nonfat Greek yogurt at the temperature of your room
- 1 packet of ranch dressing mix, powdered
- 6 slices of turkey bacon, cooked and chopped up
- 1 cup fat-free chicken broth
- 1 T fresh chopped up chives or parsley

PREPARATION

1.   Make sure that the Greek yogurt is at room temperature. After that, spray the crock pot with cooking spray and put the chicken breasts in there
2.   Take a bowl and put all of the ingredients in there except for yogurt
3.   Put the sauce on top of the chicken
4.   Cook on high for about 3.5 hours
5.   Put in the yogurt at room temperature and mix it, and then heat it for about 10 minutes or so until the sauce is warmed
6.   Shred the chicken and then put the chives and parsley on top to garnish
7.   You can serve it over miracle noodle pasta for no additional points

VEGETARIAN LASAGNA

Prep time: 20 mins
Cook time: 2.4 hours
Servings: 8
Points: 8

Ingredients:

- 1 package of whole wheat lasagna noodles, left uncooked
- 3 cups shredded reduced fat mozzarella
- 1 can diced tomatoes
- 3 Portobello mushroom caps, thinly sliced
- ½ cup liquid egg substitute
- ¼ cup fresh basil, chopped
- ½ t salt and pepper
- 1 container of fat-free ricotta
- 1 can of crushed tomatoes
- 1 can of chopped baby spinach

- 1 eggplant cut into quarters by length and sliced up thinly
- 5 cloves minced garlic
- 1 t dried oregano

PREPARATION

1. Put the egg substitute, ricotta cheese, the salt and pepper along with the oregano, and the veggies together into a bowl, mixing it
2. Mix the tomatoes and their juices, along with the basil and the garlic into a bowl
3. Put the cooking spray onto the slow cooker, and then put about a cup and a half of the tomato mixture into there, along with 5 egg noodles over this, overlapping slightly and breaking to cover
4. Then, put about half of the ricotta veggie mixture over the noodles and then pat it down firmly
5. Put 1/5 cups of the sauce on top of that and 1 cup of the mozzarella
6. Continue to do this, layering each time, with the noodles to start. You should top this with a third layer. Make sure to evenly spread the tomato sauce over the noodles, and put the last cup of mozzarella aside
7. Cook it on high for 2 hours or low for 4 hours
8. When done, put the rest of the mozzarella on top and then let it sit for about 10 minutes in order to melt the cheese.

CROCK POT CHEESY CHICKEN AND POTATOES

Prep time: 15 mins
Cook time: 6 hours
Servings: 6
Points: 7

Ingredients:

- 2 pounds of boneless, skinless chicken breasts, cut into 6 different fillets
- 1 can of cream of chicken soup, a 10.75 oz., can
- 1 cup low-fat cheddar cheese, shredded up
- 1 t paprika
- 1 pound of gold potatoes, wedged up
- 1/3 cup fat-free chicken broth
- 1 T Worcestershire sauce
- Salt and pepper for taste

PREPARATION"

1. Take the potatoes and put them into the slow cooker, seasoning them to taste
2. Season the chicken with the paprika, pepper, and the salt and put it over the potatoes
3. Whisk the soup and the broth together and put it over the chicken and the potatoes, cooking it on low for at least 6 hours
4. Transfer the chicken and potatoes to another plate and cover it with foil
5. Set the slow cooker to high heat and then put the Worcestershire and shredded cheese in there, mixing it, cooking for around 5 or so minutes until cheese melts. Stir it until blended, and then put it over the chicken and the potatoes.

SWEET TEA GLAZED PORK LOIN

Prep time: 15 minutes
Cook time: 1 hour
Servings: 8
Points: 8

Ingredients:

- 2 pounds of pork loin roast

For the glaze, get the following:

- 4 cups water
- 8 bags of black tea
- Zest from two lemons
- 1 T olive oil
- 2 cups of blackberries, divided up
- ¼ cup tea reduction, keeping the reserve from the glaze
- 1 t cornstarch
- 1 cup sugar
- 6 sprigs of thyme
- 1 T olive oil
- ½ cup of diced onions
- ¼ cup chicken broth
- 2 T cider vinegar
- Salt and pepper for the taste

PREPARATION

1. For your glaze, you should heat the water and the sugar in a saucepan, boiling this and ten adding the tea bags, thyme, and the zest, letting it steep for about 30 or so minutes
2. Strain the mixture and then heat the tea over medium heat until you get a cup of this, usually about 30-35 minutes
3. Keep ¼ cup for the sweet tea sauce
4. While this is reducing, you should heat your cock pot and then baste the pork with the glaze every 10 minutes while the tea is cooking
5. Put it in the crock pot and heat it on high for at least an hour or two
6. Sauté the onion for about 3 minutes, until it is softened, then put the vinegar and cornstarch together, with the rest of the sauce until it's thickened
7. Break down the blackberries and then mix with the sauce
8. Take the pork out and let it sit, then put the blackberry sweet tea sauce on top of that before you serve this.

CHICKEN SLOW COOKER TACOS

Prep time: 10 mins
Cook time: 4-8 hours
Servings: 4
Points: 5

Ingredients:

- 1 pound of the boneless, skinless chicken breasts
- ¼ t pepper and salt

- 2 t ground cumin
- ½ t chili powder
- 1 cup diced tomatoes
- ¼ cup chopped cilantro
- 4 taco shells
- Toppings you desire
- 1 T olive oil
- 1 t paprika
- ½ t onion powder
- ½ of a diced red onion
- 1 juiced lime
- 2 oz., of queso fresco, crumbled up

PREPARATION

1. Season the chicken with some salt and pepper, letting it sauté in the olive oil and a skillet until it's browned on every side
2. Put the cumin, chili and onion powder, paprika, and the garlic in the crock pot with the chicken, covering it
3. Cook it on low for 6-8 hours until the chicken is tender
4. Towards the end, mix the onion, cilantro, and tomato in a bowl, seasoning with lime juice and some salt and pepper
5. Remove and shred with two forks, then serve the chicken in the shells, with the toppings of choice.

SLOW COOKER CHICKEN STEW RECIPE

Prep time: 15 mins
Cook time: 6 hours
Servings: 4
Points: 5

Ingredients:

- 4-6 boneless, skinless chicken thighs
- 1 cup fat-free chicken broth
- 1 chopped head of cauliflower
- 1 can of drained artichoke hearts
- 1/3 cup of Kalamata olives, drained
- 8 cloves of minced garlic
- 1 t salt
- 1 can of diced tomatoes
- ½ cup of plain, fat-free yogurt
- 1 sliced fennel bulb
- 1 sliced red onion
- ¼ cup chopped oregano
- 2 t lemon zest
- ½ t black pepper

Direction:

1.   Spray a skillet with cooking spray and let it sit at medium high heat, browning the chicken on each side, typically taking about 5 minutes
2.   Put the chicken into the slow cooker, putting the fennel, cauliflower, olives, and onion around the chicken.
3.   Put the garlic, zest, salt and pepper, and the oregano over all of this
4.   Put the broth and tomatoes into there
5.   Cook it on high for about 4-5 hours or 6-8 on low
6.   Put the yogurt and artichokes into there and then let it cook for about another 20-30 minutes, or until they're warmed and softened.

SLOW COOKER CHEESY RISOTTO

Prep time: 20 mins
Cook time: 3-4 hours
Servings: 6
Points: 5

Ingredients:
- 1 cup short grain brown rice
- 1 cup water
- 1 diced fennel bulb
- 1/3 cup diced onions
- 1 chopped shallot
- ½ cup parmesan cheese, grated
- 2 t fennel seeds
- 1 T grated lemon zest
- 4 cups vegetable broth
- 1/3 cup dry white wine
- 2 cups of fresh-cut green beans
- 1 carrot, peeled and chopped up
- ½ cup chopped mushrooms
- 1/3 cup plain Greek yogurt
- 3 cloves minced garlic
- Salt and pepper for taste

PREPARATION
1.   Spray the inside of your slow cooker with cooking spray
2.   Crush the fennel seeds with hard bottom
3.   Mix the fennel seeds, rice, fennel that is diced, carrots and shallots, and the garlic into the slow cooker. Put the broth, a cup of water, and the wine together to combine all of this. You should cook this until rice is tender, but also chewy and the risotto is very thick and has a creamy texture, typically anywhere from 2-3.5 hours.
4.   Before you serve this, cook your green beans based on the instructions and then drain them.
5.   Turn off the slow cooker and put in the rest of the veggies, parmesan, the yogurt, lemon zest, and the pepper into there. If it is drier than expected, put a bit of water into there as it's heated and stir it into the risotto for the best results.

SLOW COOKER POT ROAST

Prep time: 15 mins
Cook time: 8
Servings: 8
Points: 5

Ingredients:

- 4 pound lean beef chuck roast, with the fat trimmed off
- 2 sliced onions
- 1 cup chopped butternut squash
- 1 t dried thyme and sage
- ½ cup strong brewed coffee
- 2 T cornstarch with 2 T water mixed
- 1 T olive oil
- ½ cup sliced carrots
- 4 cloves of minced garlic
- 1 T chopped parsley
- 2 T balsamic vinegar
- Salt and pepper for taste

PREPARATION

1. Preheat your oven to 300 and season the beef with some salt and pepper
2. Heat oil in Dutch oven and then brown the beef on all sides
3. Put this into the slow cooker and then put the veggie, spices, coffee, and vinegar together and then let it simmer. Cook it until its tender, usually about 4.5-5 hours on high or 7-8 on low.
4. Put the butternut squash and parsley in when the last 2 hours of cooking happens
5. Take the fat from the braising liquid and then put it in a saucepan, adding in the cornstarch until it creates a gravy sort of texture, usually about a minute or so. Carve the beef that you have and serve it with the gravy that you've created for the best results.

SLOW COOKER ASIAN SPICED BEANS

Prep time: 1.5 hours if using dried beans, about 20 minutes if not.
Cook time: 6 hours
Servings: 6
Points: 7

Ingredients:

- ½ cup dry package navy beans and red beans, both rinsed and drained out
- 1 pound of boneless and skinless chicken breasts, cut into cubes about ½ an inch
- 2-3 t minced garlic, more to taste
- 1 can of fat-free chicken broth
- ½ t crushed red pepper
- 4 cups cooked rice
- 3 carrots, sliced diagonally
- 2-3 t minced ginger root
- 2 T cornstarch
- 2-3 T low-sodium soy sauce

- Sliced green onions or some chopped peanuts to garnish this

PREPARATION

1. If you're going to use dry beans, put them in a saucepan and cover with about 2 inches of water, let it boil, then leave it uncovered for a couple of minutes, and then set it aside for an hour or so.
2. Drain and rinse these. You can place these soaked/canned beans, the ginger, the chicken, the carrots, and the garlic along with about 1 ¼ cups of the chicken broth into your slow cooker, stirring this
3. Cover and let it cook for about 5.5-6 hours or so
4. Mix the cornstarch with the rest of the broth and put it into the slow cooker, along with the crushed red pepper. Let it cook until it's thickened up, about 30 minutes
5. Add in the soy sauce and ten serve it over the rice, garnishing this with the green onions and the peanuts.

SLOW COOKER ROSEMARY CHICKEN

Prep time: 20 minutes
Cook time: 6 hours
Servings: 4
Points: 5

Ingredients:

- 1 roasting chicken, usually about 6 pounds, cleaned and the giblets taken out
- 1 wedged onion
- 2 t ground sage
- 2 T light butter
- 2 sliced lemons
- 3 sprigs of rosemary
- 1 t garlic powder
- Salt and pepper for taste

PREPARATION

1. Preheat your oven broiler
2. Put some salt and pepper inside the chicken cavity, then the lemon slices, half of the onion wedges, and at least 2 sprigs of rosemary
3. Put the chicken in a roasting pan, and then butter over that, and then put the sage, salt and pepper, and the garlic powder in there
4. Broil this for about 8-10 minutes or until skin is browned. If you want it darker, you should leave it in there until you have it at the desired darkness. If you want to crisp the skin, do this after you slow cook if you want
5. Put the rest of the onions and the rest of the lemon slices at the bottom of where your slow cooker is, placing the chicken over it, and then the rest of the lemons and rosemary on top of that
6. Cook it on low for about 6-8 house, or high for about 4-5 hours.

SOUPS, STEW SLOW COOKING

SLOW COOKER TACO SOUP

Serves: 4
Prep Time: 10 minutes
Cook Time: 2-3 hours

Ingredients

- 1 pound ground turkey
- 1 tablespoon coconut oil
- 1 cup tomatoes, diced
- 2 * 15 oz. cans red kidney or Romano beans, drained
- 2 cups frozen corn
- 1 yellow onion, diced
- 1 package (1 oz.) Old El Paso™ taco seasoning mix
- 4 cups beef broth
- 1 tablespoon ground cumin
- 1 tablespoon garlic powder
- 1 tablespoon onion powder
- 1 tablespoon chili powder

Toppings (Optional)

- Fresh cilantro, chopped
- Shredded cheese
- Sour cream

PREPARATION

1. Start by heating coconut oil in a large skillet over medium to high heat.
2. Brown your turkey and onion in the oil. It takes about 2-4 minutes.
3. Transfer it to the pot of your slow cooker and toss in the remaining ingredients.
4. Cook it on low for about 2-3 hours.
5. Serve with your favorite toppings.

Nutritional Information

- Calories: 391
- Fat: 16.8g
- Saturated Fat: 6g
- Carbohydrates: 30.6g
- Protein: 30g
- Dietary Fiber: 5g

Smart Points: 11

SLOW COOKER MEATBALL CHILI

Serves: 10
Prep Time: 15 minutes
Cook Time: 2-3 hours

Ingredients

- 1 pound turkey

- 1 yellow onion, chopped
- 15 ounces black beans, drained and rinsed
- 1 pound frozen corn
- 1 cup diced tomatoes
- 1 can tomato sauce
- 8 ounces mushroom, sliced
- 2 tablespoons garlic powder
- 2 tablespoons onion powder
- 1 tablespoon ground cumin
- 1 tablespoon chili powder
- Salt and pepper to taste

PREPARATION

1. Take a large mixing bowl and knead in the grounded turkey, 1 tablespoon onion powder and 1 tablespoon garlic powder.
2. Once finely kneaded, form them into meatballs and place them on the bottom of your pot.
3. Add the rest of the ingredients listed above and add the rest of the garlic powder, onion powder, cumin and chili powder.
4. Cook for 2-3 hours on high.
5. Serve hot

Nutritional Information

- Calories: 425
- Fat: 22g
- Saturated Fat: 5.6g
- Carbohydrates: 42g
- Protein: 15g
- Dietary Fiber: 8g

Smart Points: 11

HERBAL TURKEY AND VEGETABLE SOUP

Serves: 4
Prep Time: 15 minutes
Cook Time: 3-4 hours

Ingredients

- 1 pound ground turkey, diced
- 1 medium yellow onion, chopped
- 1 tablespoon olive oil
- 2 cups mushroom, sliced
- 1 green bell pepper, chopped
- 1 yellow bell pepper, chopped
- 2 medium zucchini, chopped
- 2 cups chicken broth
- 1 tablespoon garlic powder
- 1 teaspoon dried parsley
- 1 teaspoon dried thyme

- 1 teaspoon dried basil
- 1 teaspoon dried rosemary
- Salt and pepper to taste

PREPARATION
1. Take a large skillet, heat olive oil and sauté your onions for 1-2 minutes.
2. Toss in the mushrooms and bell peppers, and then cook them for 2-3 minutes.
3. Toss in the mixture to your pot.
4. On that very pan, toss in the turkey and cook it for several minutes. Make sure that it is browned.
5. Toss in the turkey to your pot as well.
6. Add the zucchini, broth, spices to your pot and cover the lid
7. Let it cook for 3-4 hours on low.
8. Season with some pepper and salt.

Nutritional Information
- Calories: 305
- Fat: 15g
- Saturated Fat: 3.2g
- Carbohydrates: 18g
- Protein: 26g
- Dietary Fiber: 1.8g

Smart Points: 5

VEGETABLE CHICKEN STEW

Serves: 4
Prep Time: 5 minutes
Cook Time: 5-6 hours

Ingredients
- 1 pound chicken breasts
- 1 pound frozen corn
- 1 pound organic frozen peas
- 2 fresh bell peppers, chopped
- 1 stalk celery, chopped
- 1 can pinto beans
- 1 can black beans
- 10 ounces tomato sauce
- 3 cups low sodium chicken broth
- 2 teaspoons garlic powder
- 2 teaspoons onion powder
- 2 teaspoons dried basil

PREPARATION
1. Toss in all of the ingredients in your slow cooker.
2. Cover the lid and let it cook for about 5-6 hours on low.
3. Serve hot.

Nutritional Information
- Calories: 604

- Fat: 15g
- Saturated Fat: 3.9g
- Carbohydrates:74g
- Protein: 45g
- Dietary Fiber: 17g

Smart Points: 15

DELICIOUS BEEF STEW

Serves: 4
Prep Time: 10 minutes
Cook Time: 8 hours

Ingredients

- 2 pounds grass-fed beef
- 1 tablespoon extra-virgin olive oil
- 2 cups beef broth
- 2 tablespoons tomato paste
- 3 carrots, peeled and chopped
- 1 yellow onion, chopped
- 2 cloves garlic, minced
- 1 cup mushrooms, chopped
- 1 cup frozen peas
- 1 piece of bay leaf
- 1 tablespoon paprika
- 1 teaspoon thyme
- 1 teaspoon Himalayan salt
- 1 teaspoon ground pepper

PREPARATION

1. Take a skillet and heat olive oil.
2. Toss in your meat and let it cook for 5 minutes.
3. Chop all of your vegetables and toss them into the pot of your slow cooker.
4. Pour in the broth and toss in the spices and tomato paste.
5. Mix them nicely until combined well.
6. Set your cooker to low and let it cook for 8 hours.
7. Taste it to make sure it is to your liking. You can also adjust by adding some cayenne, pepper, and salt.
8. Remove the bay leaf and serve.

Nutritional Information

- Calories: 544
- Fat: 33.5g
- Saturated Fat: 13g
- Carbohydrates: 60g
- Protein: 49g
- Dietary Fiber: 36g

Smart Points: 17

CREAMY CHICKEN SOUP

Serves: 4
Prep Time: 10 minutes
Cook Time: 4-6 hours

Ingredients

- 1 pound boneless, skinless chicken breast
- 4 cups low sodium chicken broth
- 4 tablespoons whole wheat pastry flour
- 2 cups unsweetened almond milk
- 1 teaspoon balsamic vinegar
- ¾ cup plain Greek Yogurt
- 1 tablespoon garlic powder
- 1 tablespoon onion powder
- Fresh parsley
- Salt and pepper to taste

PREPARATION

1. Pour the chicken broth into your slow cooker pot and whisk in the flour nicely.
2. Pour in the vinegar and the almond milk.
3. Toss in the chicken.
4. Cover it and let it cook for 4-6 hours on low.
5. Once the cooking is complete, shred the chicken using 2 forks.
6. Whisk in your Greek Yogurt, onion powder, garlic powder, pepper and salt.
7. Garnish it with some fresh parsley and serve.

Nutritional Information

- Calories: 385
- Fat: 10g
- Saturated Fat: 2.4g
- Carbohydrates: 50g
- Protein: 25g
- Dietary Fiber: 3.6g

Smart Points: 8

CREOLE CHICKEN STEW

Serves: 6
Prep Time: 15 minutes
Cook Time: 4 hours

Ingredients

- 2 pounds boneless chicken thigh, cooked
- 2 tablespoons olive oil
- 1 cup low sodium chicken broth
- 2 cups onion, chopped
- 2 cups celery, chopped
- 2 cups green bell pepper, chopped
- 6 cloves garlic, minced
- 2 cups tomatoes, chopped

- 6 ounces organic tomato paste
- 2 bay leaves
- 1 teaspoon thyme
- Fresh parsley
- Scallions
- ¼ teaspoon black pepper
- Hot sauce (optional)

PREPARATION

1. Take a large skillet and heat olive oil over medium heat.
2. Toss in the onion, bell pepper, garlic, and celery.
3. Sauté for 5-7 minutes until they are fragrant.
4. Pour the tomato paste in your vegetables and cook it again for 2 minutes
5. Pour the prepared vegetables into your slow cooker pot.
6. Toss in the chopped tomatoes, chicken broth, bay leaves, thyme, and pepper.
7. Stir everything well and mix them.
8. Add chicken in the sauce.
9. Cover and let it cook for 4 hours.

Nutritional Information

- Calories: 432
- Fat: 26g
- Saturated Fat: 7g
- Carbohydrates: 10g
- Protein: 38g
- Dietary Fiber: 2.4g

Smart Points: 6

SLOW COOKER LENTIL SOUP

Serves: 4
Prep Time: 5 minutes
Cook Time: 8 hours

Ingredients

- 2 cups dry lentils
- 4 cups vegetable stock
- 1 pound baby carrots
- 1½ cups celery, chopped
- 1 tablespoon onion powder
- ¼ cup balsamic vinegar
- Salt and pepper to taste

PREPARATION

1. Open the lid of your cooker and toss in all of the ingredients into your slow cooker pot
2. Cover and let it cook for about 8 hours on low.
3. Serve.

Nutritional Information

- Calories: 321
- Fat: 9g

- Saturated Fat: 1.3g
- Carbohydrates: 49g
- Protein: 14g
- Dietary Fiber: 14g

Smart Points: 8

TORTILLA CHICKEN STEW

Serves: 4
Prep Time: 10 minutes
Cook Time: 8 hours

Ingredients
- 1 pound chicken breasts
- 12 ounces salsa
- 1 pound frozen corn
- 1 pound bell peppers, chopped
- 3 organic corn tortilla ripped by hand
- Black olives (optional)

PREPARATION
1. Place the chicken into the bottom part of your pot and pour all of the ingredients listed above.
2. Close the lid and let it cook for about 8 hours on low.
3. Once the cooking is done, take a wooden spoon to break the chicken apart.
4. Serve with sliced black olives.

Nutritional Information
- Calories: 454
- Fat: 13g
- Saturated Fat: 3.3g
- Carbohydrates: 54g
- Protein: 32g
- Dietary Fiber: 7.3g

Smart Points: 12

ROOT VEGETABLE AND LENTIL SOUP

Serves: 2
Prep Time: 10 minutes
Cook Time: 7 hours

Ingredients
- 1 tablespoon olive oil
- 1 yellow onion, chopped
- 2 cloves garlic, minced
- 2 carrots, peeled and sliced
- 1 parsnip, peeled and sliced
- 2 celery stalks, chopped
- 1 cup brown lentils
- 4 cups vegetable broth

- 1 tablespoon reduced-sodium tamari
- Sea salt and pepper to taste

PREPARATION

1. Heat olive oil in a medium skillet over medium heat.
2. Toss in garlic, onion and sauté for about 5 minutes, and toss them into your slow cooker pot.
3. Add parsnips, carrots, lentils, celery, vegetable broth, salt, pepper, and tamari in your pot.
4. Cover it and let it cook for about 7 hours.

Nutritional Information

- Calories: 296
- Fat: 16g
- Saturated Fat: 2.3g
- Carbohydrates: 36g
- Protein: 7.4g
- Dietary Fiber: 2.8g

Smart Points: 5

ONE POT PEA CARROT SOUP

Nutrition Information

- Protein: 8.3 grams
- Carbs: 7.7 grams
- Fats: 2 grams
- Saturated Fats: 1 gram
- Sugar: 3 grams
- Fiber 2 grams
- Calories: 85

Smart Points: 2

INGREDIENTS

- Carrot (1 cup chopped)
- Garlic (1 T minced)
- Onion (.5 cups chopped fine)
- Vegetable broth (8 cups)
- Split peas (16 oz. dried)

PREPARATION

- Add all of the ingredients to a slow cooker and let them cook, covered, on a high setting for 6 hours.
- Once the ingredients are done cooking add everything else to a blender and blend well prior to serving.

LENTIL & PUMPKIN STEW

Nutrition Information

- Protein: 11 grams
- Carbs: 32 grams
- Fats: 0 grams

- Saturated Fats: 0 grams
- Sugar: .5 grams
- Fiber 10 grams
- Calories: 173

Smart Points: 4

INGREDIENTS

- Ground black pepper (to taste)
- Sea salt (to taste)
- Cilantro (1 handful chopped)
- Plain Greek yogurt (.5 cups)
- Nutmeg (1 tsp.)
- Turmeric (1 tsp.)
- Ginger (1 T ground)
- Cumin (1 T ground)
- Lime juice (1 lime)
- Tomato paste (2 T0
- Vegetable broth (4 cups)
- Onion (1 chopped fine)
- Green lentils (1 cup)
- Pumpkin (2 lbs. cubed)

PREPARATION

- Add the pepper, salt, nutmeg, turmeric, ginger, cumin, lime juice, tomato paste, vegetable broth, onion, green lentils and pumpkin tothe slow cooker.
- Cover the slow cooker and let it cook on a low heat for 6 hours.

Top each serving with plain Greek yogurt and cilantro prior to serving.

ONE POT VEGETABLE SOUP

Nutrition Information

- Protein: 4 grams
- Carbs: 28 grams
- Fats: 2 grams
- Saturated Fats: 1 gram
- Sugar: 9 grams
- Fiber 7 grams
- Calories: 131

Smart Points: 5

INGREDIENTS

- Water (2 cups)
- Vegetable broth (6 cups)
- Salt (1.25 tsp.)
- Cinnamon (2 sticks)
- Ginger (1 T minced)
- Brown Sugar (2 T)
- Onions (2 sliced)
- Olive oil (2 T)

- Butternut squash (6 lbs. sliced)

PREPARATION

- Start by making sure your oven is heated to 350 degrees F.
- Place the squash halves onto a baking sheet before placing the sheet in the oven and letting it cook 15 minutes. After it has finished baking, remove it from the stove to allow it to cool.
- As the squash cools, place a pan on the oven over a medium/high heat add in the oil and the onion and let it cook for 3 minutes before adding in the garlic, ginger and brown sugar and letting everything cook for an additional minute.
- Add the results to a slow cooker and let them cook, covered, on a low setting for 6 hours.
- Once the ingredients are done cooking, discard the cinnamon sticks and add everything else to a blender and blend well prior to serving.

SLOW COOK POTATO CHOWDER

Nutrition Information

- Protein: 9 grams
- Carbs: 28 grams
- Fats: 2.8 grams
- Saturated Fats: .5 grams
- Sugar: 1.5 grams
- Fiber 4 grams
- Calories: 170

Smart Points: 4

INGREDIENTS

- Half and half (1 cup)
- Thyme (.25 tsp. crushed)
- Bay leaf (1)
- Barley (.5 cups)
- Vegetable broth (4 cups)
- Garlic (3 cloves minced)
- Leeks (1 cup chopped)
- Carrot (1 diced)
- Potatoes (2 cups cubes)

PREPARATION

- Place all of the ingredients expect for the half and half into the slow cooker, cover it, and let it cook on a low heat for 6 hours.
- 10 minutes prior to serving, and in the half and half and let it heat, uncovered for 10 minutes.

DELICIOUS MINESTRONE SOUP

Nutrition Information

- Protein: 2 grams
- Carbs: 17 grams
- Fats: 3 grams
- Saturated Fats: 1 grams

- Sugar: 2 grams
- Calories: 250

Smart Points: 5

INGREDIENTS

- Ground black pepper (to taste)
- Sea salt (to taste)
- Parmesan cheese (3 T)
- Extra virgin olive oil (2 T)
- Potato (1 lb., diced, peeled)
- Green beans (1.5 cups chopped)
- Zucchini (1 quartered)
- Leek (1 chopped)
- Celery (1 stalk diced)
- Carrot (1 diced)
- Cannellini beans (19 oz.)
- Tomatoes (14.5 oz. diced)
- Vegetable broth (4 cups)

PREPARATION

- Add all of the ingredients except for the cheese into the slow cooker and cook, covered, on a low heat for 6 hours.
- Add the parmesan cheese prior to serving.

SLOW COOK FRENCH ONION SOUP

Nutrition Information

- Protein: 15 grams
- Carbs: 53 grams
- Fats: 8 grams
- Saturated Fats: 3 grams
- Sugar: 8 grams
- Fiber 4 grams
- Calories: 331

Smart Points: 10

INGREDIENTS

- French bread (6 slices)
- Ground black pepper (to taste)
- Sea salt (to taste)
- Goat cheese (2 oz.)
- Vegetable broth (6 cups)
- Thyme (.5 tsps. crushed)
- Thyme (3 springs)
- All-purpose flour (1 T)
- Onion (3 lbs. sliced)
- Canola oil (1 T)

PREPARATION

- Add the oil to a Dutch oven and place it over a medium heat. Add in the salt as well as the onion and let it cook for 35 minutes, stirring regularly.
- Add in the flour and let it cook for 2 minutes, stirring as needed.
- Add the onions into the slow cooker before adding in the pepper as well as the sprigs of thyme. Add in the broth and cook, covered, on a low heat for 10 hours.
- Remove the sprigs of time, plate on top of the bread and then top with the remaining ingredients as desired.

SWEET POTATO ONE POT SOUP

Nutrition Information
- Protein: 2 grams
- Carbs: 23 grams
- Fats: 1 gram
- Saturated Fats: 0 grams
- Sugar: 0 grams
- Fiber 2.6 grams
- Calories: 112

Smart Points: 2

INGREDIENTS
- Ground black pepper (to taste)
- Sea salt (to taste)
- Dry mustard (1 tsp.)
- Allspice (.5 tsp.)
- Truvia (2 packets)
- Half and half (1.5 cups)
- Sweet potatoes (4 sliced, peeled)
- Vegetable broth (2 cups)

PREPARATION
- Place the potato slices and the broth into the slow cooker, cover the slow cooker and let it cook on a medium heat for 3 hours.
- Add the results to a food processor and process well.
- Add all of the ingredients to the slow cooker, cover it, and cook at a medium heat for an additional hour.

SLOW COOK SNACKS RECIPES

DELICIOUS PLUM PUDDING WITH FRUITS

Prep Time: 50 minutes
Cook Time: 4 hours.
Servings: 12
Points: 7

INGREDIENTS

Fruits

- ¾ cup currants
- ¾ cup dried apricot
- ¾ cup dates pitted
- 145 g candied oranges
- ¾ cup orange juice
- 125 ml of masala
- 1 orange, finely grated zest

Cake

- 1 cup almond powder
- 1 tsp. ground cinnamon
- 1 tsp. of five-spices
- 1 tsp. baking powder
- ½ cup butter
- ½ cup brown sugar
- 2 eggs
- 1 ½ cup all-purpose flour

PREPARATION

Fruits

In a medium sized bowl, mix all the INGREDIENTS. Plastic wrap and soak for 12 hours while covered on with a plastic wrap.

Cake

1. Butter your loaf pan and add and line with parchment paper.
2. In a bowl, mix almond powder, spices, flour, and baking powder. Book.
3. In a medium-sized bowl, mix brown sugar and cream butter the electric mixer.
4. Beat the eggs and whisk until the mixture is homogeneous.
5. With a wooden spoon, add drained fruit and dry INGREDIENTS and stir.
6. Divide the dough into the pan and add into a slow cooker. Pour water until halfway up the pan.
7. Cook on low for 4 hours.

Nutrition Information

Calories: 260
Protein: 2g
Fat: 6g
Carbohydrates: 49g

NICE HOT CIDER CRANBERRIES

Prep time: 5 minutes
Cooking time: 20 minutes.
Servings: 6
Points: 3

INGREDIENTS

- 2 liters of cranberry juice
- Zest of 2 oranges
- 14 cloves
- 1 1/2 cup dried cranberries
- 1 c. vanilla
- 1 1/3 cup honey
- 2 cinnamon sticks

PREPARATION

1. Pour the cranberry juice into a slow cooker and set on high.
2. Stir in the orange zest, nails, cranberries, vanilla, honey, and cinnamon sticks.
3. Cook, occasionally stirring, until the casserole is heated through, about 20 minutes.

Nutrition Information

Calories: 120
Protein: 0g
Fat: 0g
Carbohydrates: 30g

HEALTHY COCKTAIL SAUSAGES

Prep time: 10 minutes
Cooking time: 2 hours.
Servings: 6
Points: 1

INGREDIENTS

- 2 ¼ cups BBQ sauce
- 1 cup packed brown sugar
- 1/2 cup ketchup
- 1 c. tablespoon Worcestershire sauce
- 1/3 cup chopped onion
- 4 packages (225 g each) cocktail sausages

PREPARATION

1. Combine and mix all INGREDIENTS in the bowl of slow cooker. Cook on low for 2 hours.

Nutrition Information

Calories: 21
Protein: 0.9g
Fat: 1.4g
Carbohydrates: 1g

REFRESHING HERBAL COMPOSITE

Prep Time: 10 minutes
Cook Time: 4hours.

Servings: 6
Points: 8
INGREDIENTS
● 3 cups brown lentils
● 1/4 cup chopped fresh parsley
● 1/4 cup curry paste
● 1 c. grated ginger
● 2 c. tablespoons chopped fresh oregano
● 2 cloves garlic, minced
● 1 c. tablespoons all-purpose flour
● 1 c. to paprika
PREPARATION
1.   Combine all INGREDIENTS in the bowl of a slow cooker 5 liters capacity; mix.
2.   Add water up to ½ inch from the edge. Cover and cook on high (HIGH) for 4 hours.

Nutrition Information
Calories: 317
Protein: 21g
Fat: 6g
Carbohydrates: 46g

SLOW COOK CHOCOLATE PUDDING

Prep Time: 30 minutes
Cook Time: 2 hours.
Servings: 8
Points: 6
INGREDIENTS
Sauce
● 2 1/4 cups brown sugar
● 1/2 cup cocoa, sifted
● 1 tbsp. cornstarch
● 4 oz. dark chocolate, coarsely chopped
● 1 1/2 cup water
● 1 1/2 cup of 35%, 15% or 5% cooking cream
● 1/2 tsp. vanilla extract
Cake
● 1 1/2 cup of all-purpose flour
● 1/2 tsp. of baking soda
● A pinch of salt
● 3/4 cup butter
● 1/2 tsp. baking powder
● 1/3 cup cocoa, sifted
● 1 egg
● 1 egg yolk
● 1 cup sugar
● 3/4 cup milk
PREPARATION

Sauce
1.   Combine cocoa, brown sugar, and starch in a saucepan. Add remaining INGREDIENTS. Bring to a boil, stirring with a whisk and simmer for 10 seconds. Transfer to slow cooker.
Cake
1.   Combine flour, baking soda, baking powder, and salt in a bowl. Set aside.
2.   Again, combine sugar and cocoa with cream butter with an electric mixer.
3.   Beat the eggs into the mixture and beat until you obtain a homogenous.
4.   Slowly add the all your dry INGREDIENTS alternating with the milk.
5.   Using a scoop or a large spoon, spread the dough over the hot chocolate sauce.
6.   Place a clean cloth over the slow cooker without touching the batter. Cover and cook for 2 hours. Remove container from slow cooker. Remove the lid and let stand for 15 minutes. Serve hot or cold.

Nutrition Information
Calories: 210
Protein: 3g
Fat: 10g
Carbohydrates: 27g

GRATIFYING STRAWBERRY PUDDING

Prep Time: 10 minutes
Cook Time: 2hours.
Servings: 6
Points: 3

INGREDIENTS
- 1 cup flour
- 1/3 cup sugar
- 1 1/2 c.Tea baking powder
- 1/2 c.Tea ground cinnamon
- 1/2 c.Salt tea
- 2 large eggs, beaten with a fork
- 2 c.Oil table
- 3 cups frozen strawberries 1 cup each: raspberries, blueberries, and strawberries
- 1/2 cup granulated sugar
- 1/2 cup water

PREPARATION
1.   Combine first 5 INGREDIENTS in a bowl.Stir.
2.   Add eggs, oil, milk and vanilla.Mix well.
3.   Pour 3.5 liters into a slow cooker
4.   Put the last 5 INGREDIENTS in a saucepan.
5.   Heat, occasionally stirring until mixture boils.
6.   Pour into slow cooker.
7.   Put 3 layers of paper towels on top of the slow cooker and cover. Cook for 2 hours at low temperature.

Nutrition Information
Calories: 140
Protein: 7g

Fat: 4.2 g
Carbohydrates: 18g

SWEET MACARONI AND CHEESE

Prep Time: 10 minutes
Cook Time: 6 hours.
Servings: 6
Points: 5

INGREDIENTS
- 225g uncooked macaroni
- 4 cups Cheddar cheese, grated, divided
- 1 can (370 ml) evaporated milk
- 1 ½ cup milk
- 2 eggs
- 1 c. teaspoon salt
- 1/2 c. pepper tea

PREPARATION
1.   Grease the inside of the bowl of the slow cooker with cooking spray and spray.
2.   In a large bowl, beat eggs, evaporated milk, and milk. Add uncooked macaroni and 3 cups shredded cheese. Transfer the bowl to the slow cooker. Sprinkle remaining grated cheese on top.
3.   Cook on low heat for 5-6 hours.
4.   Do not lift the lid during cooking.

Nutrition Information
Calories: 167
Protein: 10g
Fat: 4.5g
Carbohydrates: 21g

SLOW COOK BROWN BREAD WITH RAISINS

Prep time: 10 minutes
Cooking time: 2 hours
Servings: 3
Points: 3

INGREDIENTS
- 3 cups whole wheat flour
- 1 c.table fills baking powder
- 2 c.table molasses or corn syrup.
- 1/2 c.cinnamon tea
- 1/2 c.nutmeg tea
- 2 c.Oil table
- 1 1/2 cups water or as needed
- 1/2 cup raisins

PREPARATION
1.   Combine flour, baking powder, nutmeg, and cinnamon.Add half a cup of raisins.
2.   Add the oil, molasses, and water.Stir to moisten.

3.   Pour into a well-greased slow cooker container.
4.   Place a 5 paper towel between the lid and the container of the slow cooker to absorb excess moisture.
5.   Cook over high heat for 1 hour 45 minutes.Do not lift the lid during cooking.

Nutrition Information

Calories: 130

Protein: 3g

Fat: 0g

Carbohydrates: 29g

Fiber: 2g

TASTY ALMOND BREAD

Prep time: 5 minutes

Cooking time: 3 hours

Servings: 4

Points: 4

INGREDIENTS

- 2 cups warm water
- 1 package ofactive dry yeast
- 1 c table sugar
- 3 1/2 cups plain flour
- 1/2 tsp. teaspoon salt
- 2 tablespoons oil table
- Almond Milk

PREPARATION

1.   Preheat slow cooker to HIGH with the lid closed. Dissolve yeast in 1/2 cup warm water with sugar and put in a warm place.
2.   Put the flour in a large bowl and sprinkle with salt. Make a well in the center.
3.   When yeast is bubbling: put the rest of the water and the add oil into the flour. Stir with your fingers until all the flour is absorbed.
4.   Grease a pan and put the bread crumbs.
5.   Top with almond milk. Cover with a plate and let stand for 5 minutes in a warm place.
6.   Place on a trivet (support) in the crockpot, cover and cook for 2-3 hours.

Nutrition Information

Calories: 160

Protein: 5g

Fat: 4g

Carbohydrates: 26g

DELICIOUS CINNAMON FLAVORED OATS

Prep time: 5 minutes

Cooking time: 9 hours

Servings: 3

Points: 4

INGREDIENTS

- 2 cups of oatmeal

- 2 apples
- 1 tsp. cinnamon
- 4 cups of water

PREPARATION

1.   Pour all INGREDIENTS in a slow cooker. Do NOT stir.
2.   Cook overnight for 8 – 9 hours on low.

Nutrition Information

Calories: 160

Protein: 4g

Fat: 2g

Carbohydrates: 32g

VEGETABLES AND SIDES

VEGETABLE ENCHILADA CASSEROLE

Serves: 6
Cook Time: 4 ½ hours
SmartPoints™: 8

Ingredients:

1 ½ cups onions, minced, divided
½ cup green bell pepper, chopped
3 cloves garlic, crushed and minced
2 cups tomato puree
2 cups fire roasted tomatoes, chopped
1 teaspoon salt
1 teaspoon black pepper
2 tablespoons chili powder
2 teaspoons ground cumin
2 teaspoons cayenne pepper sauce
½ teaspoon cayenne pepper powder
1 tablespoon olive oil
1 cup carrot, shredded
1 cup zucchini, shredded
1 cup yellow squash, shredded
2 cups broccoli florets
1 cup red bell pepper, chopped
2 cups mushrooms, chopped
½ cup fresh cilantro, chopped
12 fat free tortillas
1 cup Monterey jack cheese, shredded

PREPARATION

1.   In a blender, combine ½ cup onions, green bell pepper, garlic, tomato puree, fire roasted tomatoes, salt, black pepper, chili powder, ground cumin, cayenne pepper sauce, and the cayenne pepper powder. Blend until liquefied and then set aside.
2.   Add the olive oil to a skillet over medium heat.
3.   Add the remaining onions to the skillet, along with the carrots, zucchini, and yellow squash. Sauté the mixture for 1-2 minutes.
4.   Next, add the broccoli florets, red bell pepper, and mushrooms to the skillet and sauté the mixture for 3-4 minutes.
5.   Remove the skillet from the heat and stir in the fresh cilantro.
6.   Pour on a thin layer of the blender sauce into the bottom of your slow cooker.
7.   Take each low fat tortilla and fill it with the vegetable mixture.
8.   Roll the tortilla and place it in the slow cooker, seam side down. Continue until all of the tortillas and the vegetable mixture have been used.
9.   Pour the remaining blender sauce into the slow cooker.
10.   Cover and cook on low for 4 hours.

11.   Sprinkle the cheese on top of the enchiladas, cover and cook and additional 30 minutes before serving.

Nutritional Information:

Calories 257, Total Fat 7 g, Saturated Fat 3 g, Carbs 43 g,
Fiber 13 g, Sugars 8 g, Protein 12 g

PASTA FREE VEGETARIAN LASAGNA

Serves: 8
Cook Time: 6 ½ hours
SmartPoints™: 8

Ingredients:

2 large eggplants, peeled and sliced lengthwise into ¼ inch thick pieces
1 tablespoon olive oil
1 cup red onion, diced
2 cups assorted mushrooms, sliced
5 cups fresh spinach
2 cloves garlic, crushed and minced
½ cup roasted red pepper, sliced
1 teaspoon salt
1 teaspoon black pepper
2 cups fat free ricotta cheese
1 egg, beaten
¼ cup fresh basil, chopped
1 teaspoon oregano
1 cup fresh mozzarella cheese, shredded
¼ cup fresh grated parmesan cheese
2 cups sugar free tomato sauce

PREPARATION

1.   Place the olive oil in a large skillet over medium heat.
2.   Add the red onions to the skillet and sauté for 3 minutes.
3.   Next, add in the mushrooms, spinach, and garlic. Cook, stirring frequently for 3-4 minutes.
4.   Remove the skillet from the heat and add in roasted red peppers, salt, and black pepper.
5.   In a bowl, combine the ricotta cheese, egg, basil, and oregano.
6.   Spread a thin layer of the tomato sauce into the bottom of the slow cooker.
7.   Place a layer of eggplant slices over the tomato sauce.
8.   Next, spread one half of the vegetable mixture over the eggplant.
9.   Next, place one half of the ricotta mixture over the vegetables, and follow by adding ½ cup of the sauce.
10.   Repeat another layer of eggplant, vegetables, ricotta mixture and sauce.
11.   Finish with a final layer of eggplant, followed by the remaining tomato sauce.
12.   Cover and cook on low for 6 hours.
13.   Remove the cover and sprinkle on the fresh mozzarella and parmesan.
14.   Cover and cook an additional 30 minutes before serving.

Nutritional Information:

Calories 245, Total Fat 12 g, Saturated Fat 7 g, Carbs 19 g,

Fiber 5 g, Sugars 2 g, Protein 17 g

BRILLIANT RASPBERRY BEETS

Serves: 4
Cook Time: 6 hours
SmartPoints™: 5
Ingredients:
6 cups beets, quartered
½ teaspoon salt
1 teaspoon black pepper
½ cup orange juice
¼ cup raspberry vinegar
1 tablespoon olive oil
1 tablespoon brown sugar
1 teaspoon nutmeg
1 teaspoon orange zest
PREPARATION
1.   Season the beets with the salt and black pepper.
2.   In a bowl, combine the orange juice, raspberry vinegar, olive oil, brown sugar, nutmeg, and orange zest. Whisk together until they are well combined.
3.   Place the beets in the slow cooker and then pour in the sauce and stir lightly.
4.   Cover and cook on low for 6 hours.
Nutritional Information:
Calories 145, Total Fat 3 g, Saturated Fat 1 g, Carbs 26 g,
Fiber 5 g, Sugars 20 g, Protein 4 g

CHESTNUT BRUSSELS SPROUTS

Serves: 6
Cook Time: 4 hours
SmartPoints™: 4
Ingredients:
6 cups Brussels sprouts, halved
1 tablespoon olive oil
1 tablespoon flour
½ teaspoon salt
1 teaspoon coarse ground black pepper
1 teaspoon lemon zest
1 cup onion, sliced
1 cup roasted chestnuts, chopped
½ cup parmesan cheese
1 cup vegetable stock
PREPARATION
1.   Heat the olive oil in a skillet over medium heat.
2.   Add in the Brussels sprouts and season them with the salt and black pepper.
3.   Sauté the Brussels sprouts for 1-2 minutes before sprinkling in the flour. Cook, stirring frequently for 1-2 minutes.

4. Transfer the Brussels sprouts to the slow cooker.
5. To the slow cooker, add in the lemon zest, onions, roasted chestnuts, parmesan cheese, and vegetable stock.
6. Cover and cook on low for 4 hours.
7. Stir before serving.

Nutritional Information:
Calories 122, Total Fat 4 g, Saturated Fat 1 g, Carbs 17 g,
Fiber 4 g, Sugars 2 g, Protein 6 g

EASY MAPLE MUSTARD CARROTS

Serves: 4
Cook Time: 6 hours
SmartPoints™: 2

Ingredients:
4 cups baby carrots
¼ cup Dijon mustard
¼ cup apple cider vinegar
2 tablespoons sugar free maple syrup
1 tablespoon olive oil
1 tablespoon fresh tarragon, chopped

PREPARATION
1. Place the baby carrots in the slow cooker.
2. In a bowl, whisk together the Dijon mustard, apple cider vinegar, sugar free maple syrup, olive oil, and fresh tarragon.
3. Pour the dressing over the carrots, and toss to coat them evenly.
4. Cover and cook on low for 6 hours.

Nutritional Information:
Calories 74, Total Fat 3 g, Saturated Fat 0 g, Carbs 7 g,
Fiber 2 g, Sugars 0 g, Protein 0 g

SAVORY CHERRY CORNBREAD CASSEROLE

Serves: 6
Cook Time: 4 hours
SmartPoints™: 4

Ingredients:
2 eggs
2 egg whites
1 ½ cups vegetable or chicken broth
1 teaspoon salt
1 teaspoon black pepper
1 teaspoon thyme
½ teaspoon cayenne powder
1 tablespoon olive oil
2 cloves garlic, crushed and minced
½ cup onion, chopped
½ cup celery, chopped

3 cups cornbread, cubed

1 cup cherries, pitted and chopped

PREPARATION

1.   In a bowl, whisk together the eggs, egg whites, vegetable or chicken broth, salt, black pepper, thyme, and cayenne powder. Set aside.

2.   Heat the olive oil in a skillet over medium heat.

3.   Add in the garlic, onion, and celery. Sauté for 3-5 minutes, or until the vegetables are tender.

4.   Place the cornbread, cherries, and vegetable mixture into the slow cooker.

5.   Pour the egg mixture into the cornbread and stir.

6.   Cover and cook on low for 4 hours.

Nutritional Information:

Calories 133, Total Fat 6 g, Saturated Fat 1 g, Carbs 16 g,

Fiber 1 g, Sugars 3 g, Protein 5 g

MUSHROOM PECAN WILD RICE

Serves: 8

Cook Time: 6 hours

SmartPoints™: 5

Ingredients:

2 cups wild rice

5 cups vegetable or chicken broth

1 tablespoon olive oil

¼ cup shallots, diced

2 cups leeks, sliced thin

1 cup celery, diced

2 cups mushrooms, chopped

¾ cup pecans, chopped

1 teaspoons salt

1 teaspoon black pepper

1 tablespoon fresh thyme, chopped

1 orange, zested and quartered

PREPARATION

1.   Combine the wild rice and vegetable or chicken broth in the slow cooker.

2.   Heat the olive oil in a skillet over medium heat.

3.   Add in the shallots, leeks, and celery. Sauté the mixture for 2-3 minutes.

4.   Next, add in the mushrooms and cook for 1-2 minutes longer.

5.   Transfer the vegetable mixture to the slow cooker.

6.   Add in the pecans and season the mixture with the salt, black pepper, fresh thyme, and orange zest. Mix well.

7.   Place the orange wedges in the slow cooker.

8.   Cover and cook on low for 6 hours.

9.   Remove the orange wedges before serving.

Nutritional Information:

Calories 165, Total Fat 10 g, Saturated Fat 1 g, Carbs 17 g,

Fiber 3 g, Sugars 2 g, Protein 4 g

LEMON SESAME KALE

Serves: 6
Cook Time: 6 hours
SmartPoints™: 3

Ingredients:

6 cups kale, trimmed
1 cup vegetable broth
¼ cup low sodium soy sauce
1 tablespoon sesame oil
1 tablespoon lemon juice
1 tablespoon brown sugar
1 tablespoon toasted sesame seeds
1 teaspoon lemon zest

PREPARATION

1.   Place the kale in a slow cooker.
2.   In a bowl, combine the vegetable broth, low sodium soy sauce, sesame oil, lemon juice, brown sugar, toasted sesame seeds, and the lemon zest. Whisk until well combined.
3.   Pour the sauce over the kale and stir.
4.   Cover and cook on low for 6 hours.

Nutritional Information:

Calories 77, Total Fat 3 g, Saturated Fat 1 g, Carbs 11 g,
Fiber 3 g, Sugars 4 g, Protein 3 g

VEGETARIAN RECIPES

BLACK BEAN ENCHILADAS WITH SPINACH

This recipe needs 15 minutes to prepare, 3 hours to cook and will make 8 servings.

Nutritional Information

* Protein: 26 grams
* Carbs: 30 grams
* Fats: 5 grams
* Saturated Fats: 3 grams
* Sugar: 7 grams
* Fiber 10 grams
* Calories: 217
* Smart Points: 7

INGREDIENTS

* Ground black pepper (to taste)
* Sea salt (to taste)
* Lime juice (1 lime)
* Chili powder (1 tsp.)
* Coriander (1 tsp. ground)
* Cumin (1 tsp. ground)
* Sharp cheddar cheese (1.5 cups shredded)
* Sour cream (.5 cups)
* Salsa Verde (24 oz.)
* Whole wheat tortilla (8)
* Corn (1 cup)
* Black beans (15 oz. rinsed, drained)
* Spinach (16 oz. frozen, thawed, squeezed)

PREPARATION

* Place half the total number of black beans in a large bowl and mash them prior to adding in the pepper, salt, lime juice, chili powder, coriander, cumin, other black beans, corn and spinach and mix well.
* Add half of the salsa to the slow cooker before adding the bean mixture to each tortilla and rolling tightly. Ideally all of the rolled tortillas will fit in a single layer in the slow cooker.
* Add in the rest of the salsa along with the cheese and let everything cook, covered, on a low setting for 3 hours.
* Top with jalapenos, onions, cilantro and sour cream prior to serving.

SQUASH SOUP

This recipe needs 30 minutes to prepare, 6 hours to cook and will make 12 servings.

Nutritional Information

* Protein: 4 grams
* Carbs: 28 grams
* Fats: 2 grams

- Saturated Fats: 1 gram
- Sugar: 9 grams
- Fiber 7 grams
- Calories: 131
- Smart Points: 5

INGREDIENTS

- Water (2 cups)
- Vegetable broth (6 cups)
- Salt (1.25 tsp.)
- Cinnamon (2 sticks)
- Ginger (1 T minced)
- Brown Sugar (2 T)
- Onions (2 sliced)
- Olive oil (2 T)
- Butternut squash (6 lbs. sliced)

PREPARATION

- Start by making sure your oven is heated to 350 degrees F.
- Place the squash halves onto a baking sheet before placing the sheet in the oven and letting it cook 15 minutes. After it has finished baking, remove it from the stove to allow it to cool.
- As the squash cools, place a pan on the oven over a medium/high heat add in the oil and the onion and let it cook for 3 minutes before adding in the garlic, ginger and brown sugar and letting everything cook for an additional minute.
- Add the results to a slow cooker and let them cook, covered, on a low setting for 6 hours.
- Once the ingredients are done cooking, discard the cinnamon sticks and add everything else to a blender and blend well prior to serving.

PEA SOUP

This recipe needs 5 minutes to prepare, 6 hours to cook and will make 12 servings.

Nutritional Information

- Protein: 8.3 grams
- Carbs: 7.7 grams
- Fats: 2 grams
- Saturated Fats: 1 gram
- Sugar: 3 grams
- Fiber 2 grams
- Calories: 85
- Smart Points: 2

INGREDIENTS

- Carrot (1 cup chopped)
- Garlic (1 T minced)
- Onion (.5 cups chopped fine)
- Vegetable broth (8 cups)
- Split peas (16 oz. dried)

PREPARATION

- Add all of the ingredients to a slow cooker and let them cook, covered, on a high setting for 6 hours.
- Once the ingredients are done cooking add everything else to a blender and blend well prior to serving.

MUSTARD CASSEROLE

This recipe needs 20 minutes to prepare, 6 hours to cook and will make 6servings.

Nutritional Information
- Protein: 24 grams
- Carbs: 16 grams
- Fats: 8 grams
- Saturated Fats: 3.4 grams
- Sugar: 2 grams
- Fiber 2 grams
- Calories: 245
- Smart Points: 6

INGREDIENTS
- Ground black pepper (to taste)
- Sea salt (to taste)
- Dry mustard (.5 tsp.)
- Paprika (.5 tsp.)
- Pepper (.5 tsp.)
- Garlic powder (1 tsp.)
- Scallions (6 diced)
- Fat free milk (1 cup)
- Egg whites (14)
- Mushrooms (8 oz. diced)
- Bell pepper (1 diced)
- Cheddar cheese (1 cup shredded)
- Hash browns (1 packaged frozen)

PREPARATION
- Ensure the slow cooker has been sprayed down using cooking spray to ensure nothing sticks.
- Layer in the mushrooms, onions, bell peppers and potatoes plus the cheese so that it makes two or three distinct layers.
- Combine the dry mustard, garlic powder, paprika, pepper, salt, milk and egg whites together in a mixing bowl and mix well before adding the results to the slow cooker.
- Cover the slow cooker and let it cook on a low heat for 6 hours.

LENTIL AND PUMPKIN STEW

This recipe needs 25 minutes to prepare, 6 hours to cook and will make 6servings.

Nutritional Information
- Protein: 11 grams
- Carbs: 32 grams
- Fats: 0 grams

- Saturated Fats: 0 grams
- Sugar: .5 grams
- Fiber 10 grams
- Calories: 173
- Smart Points: 4

INGREDIENTS
- Ground black pepper (to taste)
- Sea salt (to taste)
- Cilantro (1 handful chopped)
- Plain Greek yogurt (.5 cups)
- Nutmeg (1 tsp.)
- Turmeric (1 tsp.)
- Ginger (1 T ground)
- Cumin (1 T ground)
- Lime juice (1 lime)
- Tomato paste (2 T0
- Vegetable broth (4 cups)
- Onion (1 chopped fine)
- Green lentils (1 cup)
- Pumpkin (2 lbs. cubed)

PREPARATION
- Add the pepper, salt, nutmeg, turmeric, ginger, cumin, lime juice, tomato paste, vegetable broth, onion, green lentils and pumpkin to the slow cooker.
- Cover the slow cooker and let it cook on a low heat for 6 hours.
- Top each serving with plain Greek yogurt and cilantro prior to serving.

SLOW COOKER RISOTTO

This recipe needs 25 minutes to prepare, 6 hours to cook and will make 4 servings.

Nutritional Information
- Protein: 29 grams
- Carbs: 29 grams
- Fats: 11.8 grams
- Saturated Fats: 6.9 grams
- Sugar: 2 grams
- Fiber 1 grams
- Calories: 364
- Smart Points: 10

INGREDIENTS
- Ground black pepper (to taste)
- Sea salt (to taste)
- Lemon zest (1 T0
- Garlic (3 cloves minced)
- Fennel seeds (2 tsp. crushed)
- Plain Greek Yogurt (.3 cups)

- Parmesan cheese (.5 cups grated)
- Mushrooms (.5 cups chopped)
- Shallot (1 finely chopped)
- Carrot (1 peeled, chopped fine)
- Green onions (.3 cups diced)
- Green beans (2 cups cooked)
- Fennel bulb (1 cored, diced fine)
- Dry white wine (.3 cups)
- Water (1 cup)
- Vegetable broth (3 cups)
- Brown rice (1 cup)

PREPARATION

- Coat the inside of the slow cooker using cooking spray to keep things from sticking.
- Add the garlic, shallot, carrot, rice, fennel and fennel seeds into the slow cooker before adding in the wine, the water and the broth and stirring well.
- Cover the slow cooker and let it cook on a low heat for 3.5 hours.
- Prior to serving, mix in the pepper, lemon zest, yogurt, parmesan cheese, green onions, mushroom and green beans.

SWEET POTATO SOUP

This recipe needs 15 minutes to prepare, 4 hours to cook and will make 6 servings.

Nutritional Information

- Protein: 2 grams
- Carbs: 23 grams
- Fats: 1 gram
- Saturated Fats: 0 grams
- Sugar: 0 grams
- Fiber 2.6 grams
- Calories: 112
- Smart Points: 2

INGREDIENTS

- Ground black pepper (to taste)
- Sea salt (to taste)
- Dry mustard (1 tsp.)
- Allspice (.5 tsp.)
- Truvia (2 packets)
- Half and half (1.5 cups)
- Sweet potatoes (4 sliced, peeled)
- Vegetable broth (2 cups)

PREPARATION

- Place the potato slices and the broth into the slow cooker, cover the slow cooker and let it cook on a medium heat for 3 hours.
- Add the results to a food processor and process well.
- Add all of the ingredients to the slow cooker, cover it, and cook at a medium heat for an additional hour.

POTATO CHOWDER

This recipe needs 10 minutes to prepare, 6 hours to cook and will make 6 servings.

Nutritional Information

- Protein: 9 grams
- Carbs: 28 grams
- Fats: 2.8 grams
- Saturated Fats: .5 grams
- Sugar: 1.5 grams
- Fiber 4 grams
- Calories: 170
- Smart Points: 4

INGREDIENTS

- Half and half (1 cup)
- Thyme (.25 tsp. crushed)
- Bay leaf (1)
- Barley (.5 cups)
- Vegetable broth (4 cups)
- Garlic (3 cloves minced)
- Leeks (1 cup chopped)
- Carrot (1 diced)
- Potatoes (2 cups cubes)

PREPARATION

- Place all of the ingredients expect for the half and half into the slow cooker, cover it, and let it cook on a low heat for 6 hours.
- 10 minutes prior to serving, and in the half and half and let it heat, uncovered for 10 minutes.

MINESTRONE SOUP

This recipe needs 20 minutes to prepare, 6 hours to cook and will make 8 servings.

Nutritional Information

- Protein: 2 grams
- Carbs: 17 grams
- Fats: 3 grams
- Saturated Fats: 1 grams
- Sugar: 2 grams
- Fiber 5 grams
- Calories: 250
- Smart Points: 5

INGREDIENTS

- Ground black pepper (to taste)
- Sea salt (to taste)
- Parmesan cheese (3 T)
- Extra virgin olive oil (2 T)
- Potato (1 lb., diced, peeled)

- Green beans (1.5 cups chopped)
- Zucchini (1 quartered)
- Leek (1 chopped)
- Celery (1 stalk diced)
- Carrot (1 diced)
- Cannellini beans (19 oz.)
- Tomatoes (14.5 oz. diced)
- Vegetable broth (4 cups)

PREPARATION

- Add all of the ingredients except for the cheese into the slow cooker and cook, covered, on a low heat for 6 hours.
- Add the parmesan cheese prior to serving.

FRENCH ONION SOUP

This recipe needs 45 minutes to prepare, 10 hours to cook and will make 6 servings.

Nutritional Information

- Protein: 15 grams
- Carbs: 53 grams
- Fats: 8 grams
- Saturated Fats: 3 grams
- Sugar: 8 grams
- Fiber 4 grams
- Calories: 331
- Smart Points: 10

INGREDIENTS

- French bread (6 slices)
- Ground black pepper (to taste)
- Sea salt (to taste)
- Goat cheese (2 oz.)
- Vegetable broth (6 cups)
- Thyme (.5 tsp crushed)
- Thyme (3 springs)
- All-purpose flour (1 T)
- Onion (3 lbs. sliced)
- Canola oil (1 T)

PREPARATION

- Add the oil to a Dutch oven and place it over a medium heat. Add in the salt as well as the onion and let it cook for 35 minutes, stirring regularly.
- Add in the flour and let it cook for 2 minutes, stirring as needed.
- Add the onions into the slow cooker before adding in the pepper as well as the sprigs of thyme. Add in the broth and cook, covered, on a low heat for 10 hours.
- Remove the sprigs of time, plate on top of the bread and then top with the remaining ingredients as desired.

SLOW COOKER COOKING TIPS

1.   Pick the correct cut: Chuck broils, short ribs, pork shoulders and sheep shanks (think greasy and harder meats) turn out to be meltingly delicate with the damp, low warmth of a slow cooker. Less fatty slices of pork tenderloin tend to dry out. In like manner, dim meat chicken — thighs, drumsticks, and so forth — will stay juicier than white meat bosoms.

2.   Keep the top shut: Each look you take amid the cooking procedure will add an extra 15 to 20 minutes of cooking time. Also, check the inclination to mix; it's generally a bit much and has a tendency to slow down the cooking.

3.   Watch over your vessel: The fired embed in a slow cooker can break if presented to sudden temperature shifts. As such, don't put a hot artistic embed straightforwardly on a frosty counter; put down a dishtowel first. The same goes for utilizing a filled embeds you've stored overnight in the icebox: Let it come to room temperature before placing it in a preheated base.

4.   Cut down fat: For luxurious sauces and flavors, pause for a moment or two and cut the abundance fat from the meat. Avoid this progression and you chance winding up with sleek, oily cooking fluid. Whenever possible, evacuate chicken skin as well.

5.   Set the warmth level: A general dependable guideline is that cooking on the low setting (170 degrees F for most models) takes about twice the length cooking on high (280 degrees F on general models). Remember that a few cuts of meat and formulas are more qualified to one setting over the other. (See tips on picking the correct cut, above.)

6.   Include dairy after everything else: Sour cream, drain, and yogurt tend to separate in the slow cooker, so blend them in amid the most recent 15 minutes of cooking.

Nancy Huckabee

Bonus Freestyke Instant Pot Recipes from my next book

Zero Point Food

• Boneless skinless turkey breast

• Thin sliced deli chicken breast

• Ground lean chicken

• Fresh, frozen, and canned beans and lentils that are packed without oil or sugar (Lentils, pinto beans, chickpeas, black beans, kidney beans, split peas, soy beans, and more)

• Boneless skinless chicken breast

• Thin sliced deli turkey breast

• Ground lean turkey

• Canned fish that is packed in water or brine (i.e. canned tuna or canned salmon in water)

• All fish and shellfish (this does not include smoked or dried fish)

• Tofu and smoked tofu

• Eggs

• Quorn fillets, ground Quorn, and Quorn pieces (meat substitute)

• Plain soy yogurt

INSTANT POT BEEF RECIPES

6PTS INSTANT POT MEXICAN BEEF

Ready in 50 minutes,
6 servings
Freestyle Points value per serving: 6

Ingredients

- 3 pounds' boneless beef short ribs sliced into cubes
- ½ cup chili powder
- 2 teaspoons salt
- 1 tablespoon fat
- 1 medium onion, thinly sliced
- 2 tablespoon tomato paste
- 5 garlic cloves, well peeled and smashed
- ½ cup roasted tomato salsa
- ½-1 cupbone broth
- 1 teaspoonRed Boat Fish Sauce
- black pepper, freshly ground
- ½ cup minced cilantro
- 2 radishes, thinly sliced

Instructions

1. Combine the cubed beef, chili powder, and salt in a large bowl.
2. Bring pot to medium heat and when the fat melts, add the onions then sauté until soft.
3. Stir in tomato paste and garlic, and cook until fragrant or 30 seconds.
4. Add in the seasoned beef then pour in the salsa, fish sauce and stock.
5. Tight lid the pot and cook on high heat until high pressure is reached. Afterwards, lower the heat to maintain high pressure for about 30 minutes. Release pressure naturally for 15 minutes.
6. Unlock the lid, season with salt and pepper to taste and serve.

Nutrition information

Calories: 209.5
Carbohydrates: 6.8g
Fats: 13.4g
Proteins: 15.1g

7PTS MAPLE SMOKED BRISKET

Ready in 1 hr. 30 minutes
8 servings
Freestyle Points value per serving: 7

Ingredients

- 1 lb. beef brisket
- 1-2 tablespoons maple, date, or coconut sugar,
- 2 teaspoons sea salt, smoked
- 1 teaspoon black pepper

- 1 teaspoon mustard powder
- 1 teaspoon onion powder
- ½ teaspoon smoked paprika
- 2 cups bone broth
- 3 fresh thyme sprigs

Instructions

1. Withdraw the brisket from refrigerator 30 minutes before cooking. Dry it with paper towels and set aside.
2. Combine the maple sugar, pepper, smoked sea salt, onion powder, mustard powder, and smoked paprika.Coat the meat with the mixture on all sides.
3. Add to the Instant Pot and allow it to fry for 2-3 minutes until golden brown. Turn the brisket and add the broth, thyme and liquid smoke. Scrape any browned bits at the bottom and then cover with the lid.
4. Allow to cook for 50 minutes and release steam naturally. Withdraw the brisket from the pot cover with foil and set aside. Slice the brisket and serve it.

Nutrition information

Calories: 542.9
Carbohydrates: 30.3g
Fats: 24g
Proteins: 45.6g

5PTS FREESTYLE SPICY BRAISED BEEF

Time: 90 mins
Number of servings: 4
Freestyle Points value per serving: 5

Ingredients:

- Two pounds chopped into 3-inch pieces eye of round beef, without fat four cloves garlic half of medium onion Juice of one lime.
- Two tbsps. chipotles in adobo sauce
- One tbsp. ground oregano
- One tbsp. ground cumin
- One cup water
- Two tsp kosher salt
- Three bay leaves
- One tsp olive oil
- Pinch of ground cloves
- Black pepper to taste

Directions:

• Season the beef with salt and pepper. Pour oil into your Instant Pot, place meat and select "Sauté" function. Cook meat until it's browned.
• Blend lime juice, onion, garlic, water, chipotle, oregano, and cloves in your blender.
• Pour that blended mixture into the pot and mix bay leaves. Select "Manual" function to cook on high pressure for one hour.
• Use natural pressure release method.
• Remove the meat from the pot then shred it. And mix this shredded beef with cooking liquid.

• Serve and enjoy!

8PTS TENDER BEEF BOURGUIGNON

Ready in 1 hour,
6 servings
Freestyle Points value per serving: 8

Ingredients

- 4-6 strips smoked bacon, chopped
- 2 lbs. chuck beef sliced
- 6 tablespoons flour, all purpose
- 1 tablespoon sea salt
- ½ teaspoon black pepper
- 3 tablespoon butter
- 1 lb. carrots, cut into thin chunks
- 5 garlic cloves, chopped
- 2 sliced yellow onions
- 1 lb. quartered fresh mushrooms
- 1 bay leaf
- 1 teaspoon fresh thyme leaves
- 3-4 cups red wine
- 2 cups stock or beef broth
- 1 tablespoon tomato paste

Instructions

1. Make Marinade. Dry the beef with paper towel.
2. Marinade the meat in 4 cups of red wine, salt and pepper. Allow to stay overnight.
3. Drain the beef but keep the wine, dry the beef with a paper towel and put the chunks in a bowl. Coat all sides generously with flour, salt, and pepper, set aside.
4. On the Instant Pot select "Saute" and add in the chopped bacon and the meat pieces. If possible, cook the in batches. Afterwards, withdraw them and set aside.
5. Melt the butter and add carrots, garlic and onions. Sauté until onions are softened. Add in mushrooms and sauté for a minute.
6. Add the reserved wine, thyme and bay leaf. Allow to 'simmer' for about 3 minutes. Add in the beef, beef broth and tomato paste. Stir well.
7. Tightly close with lid and ensure the vent valve is closed. Select MEAT setting (30 minutes). Add any remaining flour to butter to make a roux.
8. Let the pressure release naturally and add the roux to thicken the sauce. Serve over any carb

Nutrition information

Calories: 461
Carbohydrates: 12g
Fats: 18g
Proteins: 49g

6PTS FREESTYLE FAST BEEF MEATBALLS

Time: 20 mins

Number of servings: 4
Freestyle Points per serving: 6
Ingredients:
- One pound ground beef
- Two crumbled bread slices
- Two chopped carrots
- Two cups pasta sauce
- Two cups water
- One chopped onion
- One beaten egg
- Half tsp garlic salt
- Salt and pepper to taste

Directions:
1. Take a mixing bowl and mix ground beef, egg, crumbled bread, onion, carrots, garlic salt, salt, and pepper.
2. Make meatballs from that mixture and set them aside.
3. Pour water and pasta sauce into your Instant Pot and stir well.
4. One by one add meatballs in the pasta sauce mixture.
5. Seal pot with the lid, select "Manual" and cook on high pressure for five minutes.
6. Allow release pressure naturally.
7. Serve meatballs with pasta, rice, and enjoy!

7PTS VEGETABLE STUFFED PEPPERS WITH BEEF

Time: 30 mins
Number of servings: 4
Freestyle Points per serving: 7
Ingredients:
- One pound ground beef
- One cup brown rice
- Four bell peppers
- One diced tomato
- One can tomato sauce
- One egg
- One chopped onion
- One cup shredded mozzarella cheese
- Half tsp dried parsley
- Half tsp garlic powder
- Half tsp oregano
- Salt and pepper to taste

Directions:
1. Take a mixing bowl and mix ground beef, rice, egg, tomato, onion, parsley, oregano, salt, and pepper.
2. Slice off the bell peppers tops. Then stuff meat mixture into the bell peppers.
3. Pour water and half of tomato sauce in your Instant Pot. Then place a trivet in the pot and place stuffed peppers on top.
4. Now pour all remaining tomato sauce over the top of peppers.

5.	Seal the pot with the lid and select "Manual" function for fifteen minutes.
6.	Use natural pressure release. Open the lid carefully and add mozzarella cheese on the top of peppers.
7.	Close the lid again just for a few seconds, until cheese melted.
8.	Serve immediately and enjoy!

7PTS PRESSURE COOKER POT ROAST

Ready in 1 hr. 45 minutes,
6 servings
Freestyle Points value per serving: 7

Ingredients
- 3 lbs. boneless chuck roast
- 1/2 tablespoon ghee
- 1/2 teaspoon black pepper
- 1/2 teaspoon salt
- 1 yellow onion, chopped
- 2 clove garlics, minced
- 1 tablespoon tomato paste
- 2 cups beef broth
- 1 cup chicken broth
- 1/4 cup red wine
- 1 tablespoon Worcestershire sauce
- 2 lbs. red potatoes, sliced into thin chunks
- 2 lbs. carrots, chopped
- 5-6oz white mushrooms, sliced in half
- salt and pepper

Instructions:
1.	Season the roast with salt and pepper. Add in the ghee to the instant pot and fry for about 2 minutes and then add the roast. Allow all sides to brown for about 6 minutes each
2.	Withdraw the roast and put aside. Add in the onion and fry for about 4 minutes until softened and stir often then add the garlic and tomato paste, stir together for 30 seconds until aromatic.
3.	Add in the broths, wine, and Worcestershire sauce. Combine well by stirring and bring to a simmer. Add the roast and any juices.
4.	Cover the pot and set it on high pressure for 45 minutes. Once finished. Afterwards, release pressure naturally.
5.	Withdraw the lid and transfer the roast to a baking sheet, set aside.
6.	Add the potatoes, mushrooms and carrots to the Instant Pot, cover with the lid, and bring pressure to high for 6 minutes. Meanwhile, transfer the roast to the oven and broil for 4 minutes, remove again and transfer it to a cutting board.
7.	Release pressure form Instant Pot once the vegetables are cooked. Transfer the vegetables to the baking sheet using a slotted spoon.
8.	Place the vegetables in the oven and then broil for 5 minutes until browned. Slice the roast and place it on a platter and add the vegetables to the same platter. Pour some of the simmered liquid over the roast and vegetables. Serve immediately with the sauce.

Nutrition information

Calories: 256, Carbohydrates: 1g, Fats: 16g, Proteins: 25g

8PTS GRAIN FREE MEATBALLS AND SAUCE

Ready in 3-4 hours,
8-10 servings
Freestyle Points value per serving: 8

Ingredients:

- 2 eggs
- pound organic beef, ground
- 4-5 tablespoons, fruit-sweetened grape jelly
- 1/2 cup , organic
- 1/2 teaspoon pepper, ground
- 1/2 teaspoon Spanish paprika
- 1/4 teaspoon chili powder
- 1 teaspoon ground garlic salt
- 1/4 cuptapioca flour or arrowroot

Instructions

1. Heat oven to about 350
2. Combine the beef, pepper, eggs, garlic salt and tapiocastarchin a mixing bowl
3. Make small golf ball sized meatballs with the mixture and transfer to a baking sheet
4. Bake until browned or about 25 minutes.
5. Transfer the baked meatballs to crockpot, add chili sauce, paprika, grape jelly, and chili powder.
6. Cook on low heat for 2-4 hours, occasionally checking. Serve with any of your favorite greens or over rice.
7. NOTE: When an Instant Pot is used, you don't have to bake the meatballs in advance.

Nutrition information

Calories: 291.2
Carbohydrates: 33.6g
Fats: 9.5g
Proteins: 19.4g

6PTS PRESSURE COOKER TEXAS RED CHILI

Ready in 1 hour, 6 servings,
Freestyle Points value per serving: 6

Ingredients

- 1 tablespoon vegetable oil
- 4-5 pounds' beef chuck roast, chopped 2 inch cubes
- ½ tablespoon kosher salt
- 2 onions, diced
- 3 cloves garlic, minced
- 2 minced chipotles with sauce
- 1/2 teaspoon kosher salt
- 1 teaspoon chili powder

- ½ cup cumin
- 2 teaspoons Mexican oregano
- 1 cup coffee
- 14 ounces can of crushed tomatoes
- Salt and pepper to taste

Instructions

1. Brown the beef: Heat the oil in the cooker pot over medium-high heat for 30 seconds. Sprinkle the beef with salt and then brown in two to three batches. Brown each batch on one side, about five minutes.
2. Add in the onions and 1/2 teaspoon of kosher salt to the cooker. Fry the onions for about 5 minutes until softened while scraping with a spoon to remove any stuck bits on the bottom. Add the garlic cloves and chipotle and then fry for one minute. Add the chili powder, oregano and cumin. Allow to cook for one minute and then stir the spices into the onions.
3. Pour the beef and any juices into the cooker, and then add the crushed tomatoes. Stir until the beef is completely coated in tomatoes and spices.
4. Shut the cooker tightly, bring the high heat and maximum pressure. Cook for 25 minutes and then release pressure naturally, about 15 minutes and then remove the lid.
5. Add salt to reduce chili bitterness. Serve the chili straight up.

Nutrition information

Calories: 225
Carbohydrates: 7g
Fats: 16g
Proteins: 14g

CPSIA information can be obtained
at www.ICGtesting.com
Printed in the USA
LVHW021006120621
689863LV00005B/42